Children's Mental Health

Problems and Services

A Report by the Office of Technology Assessment

Denise M. Dougherty, Study Director, OTA

Leonard M. Saxe, Boston University, Principal Author

with Theodore Cross, Boston University, and

Nancy Silverman, Boston University

Duke Press Policy Studies
Duke University Press   Durham

D0521507

Published by Duke University Press
6697 College Station
Durham, North Carolina 27708
First Duke University Press edition, 1987.
LCC 86-600539
ISBN 0-8223-0796-0 (archival quality paper, casebound)
ISBN 0-8223-0815-0 (paperback)

Reprinted by arrangement with the Office of Technology Assessment, Congress of the United States, Washington, D.C. 20510.

Publisher's note. Undertaken by the Office of Technology Assessment at the request of the U.S. Senate Appropriations Committee, and made public in December 1986. It is the intention of Duke University Press to make this report available to a wider audience of libraries, concerned citizens, and professionals.

Clothbound editions of Duke University Press books are printed on acid-free paper, and bound with materials selected for strength and durability. Duke University Press paperbacks, while suitable for personal use, are not manufactured to perform to library archival standards.

Printed and bound in the United States of America

Office of Technology Assessment

The Office of Technology Assessment (OTA) was created in 1972 as an analytical arm of Congress. OTA's basic function is to help legislative policymakers anticipate and plan for the consequences of technological changes and to examine the many ways, expected and unexpected, in which technology affects people's lives. The assessment of technology calls for exploration of the physical, biological, economic, social, and political impacts that can result from applications of scientific knowledge. OTA provides Congress with independent and timely information about the potential effects—both beneficial and harmful—of technological applications.

Requests for studies are made by chairmen of standing committees of the House of Representatives or Senate; by the Technology Assessment Board, the governing body of OTA; or by the Director of OTA in consultation with the Board.

The Technology Assessment Board is composed of six members of the House, six members of the Senate, and the OTA Director, who is a non-voting member.

OTA has studies under way in nine program areas: energy and materials; industry, technology, and employment; international security and commerce; biological applications; food and renewable resources; health; communication and information technologies; oceans and environment; and science, education, and transportation.

The views expressed in this background paper do not necessarily represent those of the Technology Assessment Board, OTA Advisory Council, or individual members thereof.

OTA Project Staff
Children's Mental Health:
Problems and Services

Roger C. Herdman, Assistant Director, OTA
Health and Life Sciences Division

Clyde J. Behney, Health Program Manager

Denise M. Dougherty, Study Director
Kerry Britten Kemp, Health and Life Sciences
Division Editor
Brad Larson, Research Assistant (Until June 1986)
Beckie Berka, Research Assistant (Until June 1986)
Laura T. Mount, Research Assistant
Virginia Cwalina, Administrative Assistant
Diann G. Hohenthaner, PC Specialist/
Word Processor
Carol A. Guntow, Secretary/Word Processor
Specialist
Karen Davis, Clerical Assistant

Contractors
Leonard M. Saxe, Boston University,
Principal Author,
with Theodore Cross, Boston University,
and Nancy Silverman, Boston University
Walter F. Batchelor, Boston University

Foreword

Within the past several years, several important mental health problems of children have been the focus of congressional attention. The incidence of adolescent suicide, physical and sexual abuse of young children, alcohol and drug abuse by children, and psychiatric hospitalization of children and adolescents have been the focus of debate on the need for an appropriateness of mental health services. This background paper indicates that although there are no simple answers to when and what type of mental health services are necessary, the need for a mental health system response, coordinated with activities of other service systems, seems well documented.

This background paper was requested by Senators Mark O. Hatfield and Daniel K. Inouye through the Senate Appropriations Committee. Its development was guided by a panel of experts chaired by Dr. Lenore Behar. The key contractor was Dr. Leonard Saxe and his colleagues at Boston University. Key OTA staff for the background paper were Denise Dougherty and Kerry Kemp.

JOHN H. GIBBONS
Director

Contents

Contents—continued

Contents—continued

Tables

Contents—continued

Figures

Chapter 1
Summary and Policy Implications

Summary and Policy Implications

INTRODUCTION

Mental health problems are a source of suffering for children, difficulties for their families, and great loss for society. Though such problems are sometimes tragic, an even greater tragedy may be that **we currently know more about how to prevent and treat children's mental health problems than is reflected in the care available.** This background paper was requested by the Senate Appropriations Committee through Senators Mark O. Hatfield and Daniel K. Inouye, who expressed special interest in learning the extent to which the mental health field has reached a consensus on the appropriate treatments and treatment settings for responding to the mental health needs of our Nation's children. It examines the nature of children's mental health problems, the mental health services available to aid disturbed children, and the Federal role in providing services.

The problems that affect children's mental health range from transient conditions in a child's environment to diagnosable mental illnesses. Mental health problems that meet the diagnostic criteria contained in the third edition of the American Psychiatric Association's *Diagnostic and Statistical Manual*, the "DSM-III,"[1] are identified in this background paper by the terms *mental disorders*, *diagnosable mental disorders,* and *DSM-III disorders*. Typically, the existence of a DSM-III disorder is necessary for obtaining third-party reimbursement for mental health services. Other terms like *mental health problems* and *disturbed children* refer in this background paper not only to DSM-III disorders, but also to children's mental health problems more generally—i.e., to disturbed self-esteem, developmental delays, and other subclinical problems that children may experience as a result of environmental stress. Currently, services for problems other than DSM-III disorders are seldom eligible for third-party payment.

Interventions to prevent and treat children's mental health problems are as diverse as children's problems. This background paper considers several issues related to the provision of mental health services for children, emphasizing in particular, psychiatric hospitalization—the most restrictive and costly form of treatment.

Although serious policy questions remain concerning the provision of adequate, appropriate, and cost-effective mental health services to children, several conclusions can be drawn from this background paper:

- **Many children do not receive the full range of necessary and appropriate services to treat their mental health problems effectively.** However, the precise nature of the gap between what mental health services are being provided to children and what should be provided is not clear.
- **A substantial theoretical and research base suggests that, in general, mental health interventions for children are helpful,** although it is often not clear what intervention is best for particular children with particular problems. Most important for the focus of this paper, the effectiveness of psychiatric hospitalization for treating childhood mental disorders has not been studied systematically.
- **Although there seem to be shortages in all forms of children's mental health care, there is a particular shortage of community-based services, case management, and coordination across child service systems**—all of which are necessary to provide a comprehensive and coordinated system of mental health care throughout the country. Models for providing community-based continuums of mental health care exist, and preliminary evidence suggests that such continuums can be effective; these deserve careful and large-scale trials with systematic evaluation.

---

[1]At the time this background paper was being prepared, DSM-III was being revised by the American Psychiatric Association. The new version will be known as DSM-III-R.

Available epidemiologic data indicate that at least 12 percent, or 7.5 million, of the Nation's approximately 63 million children suffer from emotional or other problems that warrant mental health treatment—and that figure may be as high as 15 percent, or 9.5 million children. These epidemiologic data, while not based on systematic, recent national studies, are widely accepted and give some indication of the magnitude of children's mental health care needs.

Like estimates of children's mental health needs, information about mental health care utilization by children is somewhat dated. The most recent mental health care utilization data available[2] show that less than 1 percent of the Nation's children, or 100,000 children, receive mental health treatment in a hospital or residential treatment center (RTC) in a given year, and perhaps only 5 percent, or 2 million children, receive mental health treatment in outpatient settings (see figure 1). Using these data, OTA estimates that from 70 to 80 percent of children in need may not be getting appropriate mental health services.

It is not always clear why children do not receive needed mental health services. Some children may not receive services because of the stigma attached to having a mental disorder. Other children may not receive services because the services are not available in their communities. Still others may not receive services because their families cannot afford them. Using the most recent data available (1977), OTA estimates that 14 million of the Nation's approximately 63 million children may not have any private health insurance. Furthermore, the insurance that is available for mental health problems is generally restricted to treating diagnosable mental disorders, is significantly less generous than insurance for other disorders, and covers outpatient care less generously than inpatient care.

To the extent that treatment decisions are based on service system or financial considerations, inappropriate mental health care may be given. Some children may be undertreated (e.g., be given outpatient treatment when they require hospital

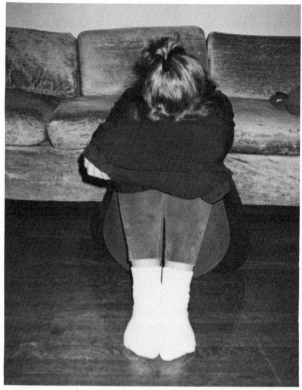

Photo credit: OTA

Mental health problems are a source of suffering for children, difficulties for their families, and great loss for society.

or other residential care), and some children may be given overly intensive treatments (e.g., be treated in a psychiatric hospital when they could be treated without 24-hour medical supervision). Unfortunately, the data needed to understand precisely which children and problems should be treated in different settings have not been collected.

OTA's finding that many children with mental health problems do not receive needed care is, perhaps disappointingly, wholly consistent with the findings of commissions and study groups over the past half century. In recent years, as knowledge of the effects of children's mental health problems has grown, the urgency of addressing these problems has increased. Providing the most appropriate mental health services for children is a daunting task. The immensity of the difficulties, however, should not restrain specific efforts to improve current policy and practice.

---

[2]The most recent year for which mental health service utilization data are available is 1980, or in some cases, 1981.

Figure 1.—Estimated Numbers of Children Who Need and Who Receive Mental Health Services, 1980[a]

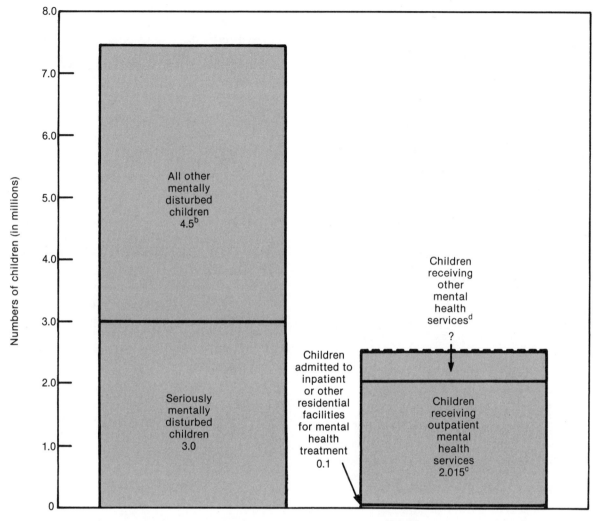

[a]Excludes prevention.

[b]The President's Commission on Mental Health indicated in 1978 that as many as 15 percent of the Nation's children—which would translate to 9.5 million of the total 63.8 million children in 1980—were in need of mental health services (excluding prevention) (514). Gould, Wunsch-Hitzig, and Dohrenwend have since estimated that 11.8 percent—or 7.5 million—of the Nation's children have mental health disturbances (248). A number of factors account for differences in estimates of children in need of mental health services (see text).

[c]Extrapolations from surveys of adults suggest that the number of children receiving outpatient mental health services could be as high as 4.02 million. A firmer estimate awaits the results of NIMH's epidemiologic catchment area survey for children (see text).

[d]Partial hospitalization, etc.

SOURCES: **Seriously mentally disturbed children in need of services:** President's Commission on Mental Health, *Report to the President From the President's Commission on Mental Health,* vol. 1 (Commission Report) (Washington, DC: U.S. Government Printing Office, 1978); and J. Knitzer, *Unclaimed Children* (Washington, DC: Children's Defense Fund, 1982).

Total number of mentally disturbed children in need of services: President's Commission on Mental Health, *Report to the President From the President's Commission on Mental Health,* vol. 1 (Commission Report) (Washington, DC: U.S. Government Printing Office, 1978); and M.S. Gould, R. Wunsch-Hitzig, and B. Dohrenwend, "Estimating the Prevalence of Childhood Psychopathology: A Critical Review," *Journal of the American Academy of Child Psychiatry* 20:462, 1981.

Children receiving inpatient or other residential mental health services: U.S. Department of Health and Human Services, Public Health Service, Alcohol, Drug Abuse, and Mental Health Administration, National Institute of Mental Health, *Mental Health, United States, 1985,* C.A. Taube and S.A. Barrett (eds.), DHHS Pub. No. (ADM) 85-1378 (Rockville, MD: 1985).

Children receiving outpatient mental health services: Adapted from U.S. Department of Health and Human Services, Public Health Service, National Center for Health Statistics, *National Medical Care Utilization and Expenditure Survey, Data Report No. 5,* "Utilization and Expenditures for Ambulatory Mental Health Care During 1980," DHHS Pub. No. 84-20000 (Washington, DC: U.S. Government Printing Office June 1984).

ORGANIZATION OF THIS BACKGROUND PAPER

The remainder of this chapter summarizes this background paper and considers policy implications. The nine remaining chapters of this background paper provide additional detail on children's mental health problems and services. The chapters are organized in five sections (see figure 2).

Part I describes efforts to assess children's mental health problems. Chapter 2 links conclusions of past study commissions about the incidence and prevalence of mental and emotional problems in children to current estimates and notes the similarities between the current situation and what were identified as problems decades ago.

Part II reviews children's mental disorders and the interrelationships of children's mental health problems and environmental conditions. Chapter 3 presents mental disorders in terms of the diagnostic categories in DSM-III. Chapter 4 considers factors in a child's family and psychosocial environment that may cause or exacerbate certain mental health problems and that may need to be considered in designing services.

Part III focuses on various approaches to treating or preventing certain children's mental health problems. Chapter 5 describes the primary therapies: individual psychotherapy based on psychodynamic, behavioral, and cognitive models; group therapy; family therapy; milieu therapy; crisis intervention; and psychopharmacological (drug) therapy. Chapter 6 describes mental health treatment settings, including hospital inpatient settings, RTCs, day treatment or partial hospitalization, and outpatient settings. Chapter 7 provides an overview of the mental health services provided to children involved in the educational, health care, child welfare, and juvenile justice systems. That chapter also describes programs aimed at preventing mental health problems and integrating mental health with other services.

Part IV examines the effectiveness of interventions used to treat and prevent children's mental health problems. Chapter 8 summarizes the research on effectiveness of the specific therapies discussed in chapter 5. Chapter 9 summarizes the research on effectiveness of treatment in mental health and other settings and the effectiveness of prevention programs. Efforts to integrate mental health and other services have not yet been evaluated.

Part V analyzes the present Federal policies aimed at alleviating children's mental health problems. Chapter 10 describes a number of Federal programs that have a direct or indirect effect on children's mental health.

SUMMARY AND POLICY IMPLICATIONS

Children's Mental Health Problems

At least 7.5 million children in the United States—representing approximately 12 percent of the Nation's 63 million children under 18—are believed to suffer from a mental health problem severe enough to require mental health treatment. The actual number of children suffering from mental disorders that meet the diagnostic criteria of DSM-III is unknown, but a fairly precise estimate will be possible with the conduct of a National Institute of Mental Health (NIMH) epidemiologic survey of children similar to that completed recently for adults. In addition to children who have diagnosable mental disorders, some children are at risk for mental suffering and disability because of environmental risk factors such as poverty, inadequate care, parental alcoholism, or divorce. These children may also benefit from mental health services.

Mental health problems of children are in many respects unlike those of adults and are much more difficult to identify. Distinguishing between normal aspects of a child's development and mental health problems that may worsen if not treated is a difficult task for parents, teachers, physicians, and mental health care professionals.

Figure 2.—Organization of This Background Paper

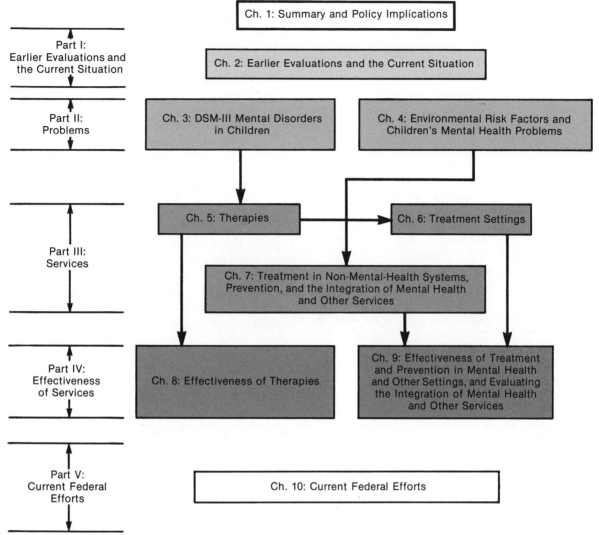

SOURCE: Office of Technology Assessment, 1986.

According to DSM-III, children may be afflicted by so-called childhood-onset mental disorders (meaning the disorder is usually manifest first in childhood) or by other disorders whose onset is not restricted to childhood. DSM-III groups mental disorders that have their onset in childhood by the area of functioning that is most impaired:

- intellectual disorders (mental retardation);
- developmental disorders (pervasive and specific developmental disorders);
- behavior disorders (attention deficit disorder and conduct disorder);
- emotional disorders (anxiety disorders, other emotional disorders of childhood or adolescence); and
- psychophysiological disorders (stereotyped movement disorders, eating disorders, and other disorders with physical manifestations).

Other mental disorders that affect children, but which more commonly begin in adulthood, include organic mental disorders; substance use disorders; schizophrenic disorders; affective disorders such as major depression; adjustment disorders; and a number of other disorders.

This background paper does not consider intellectual or developmental childhood-onset disorders except as they interrelate with other problems requiring mental health services. This exclusion reflects in part the specific wording of the request from the Senate Appropriations Committee and in part the fact that the causes, treatment, and treatment goals in the case of intellectual/developmental disorders differ from those associated with other mental disorders.

For the most part, the causes of mental disorders are unknown. However, some environmental factors, particularly psychosocial ones, pose significant risks for children's mental health.

Environmental factors that pose risks to children's mental health include poverty; parental psychopathology (e.g., schizophrenia or alcoholism); maltreatment; a teenage parent; premature birth; parental divorce; and serious childhood physical illness. These factors rarely occur in isolation and frequently interact with other aspects of a child's family, educational, and social environment. Although environmental factors do not necessarily result in mental disorders that meet the diagnostic criteria of DSM-III, they can cause maladjustment and place a child at risk for later and potentially more serious problems.

The consequences of mental health problems in children can be mild and transitory or severe and longstanding. Children with the most severe problems may be unable to function in either their home or school environments and may be dangerous to either themselves or others. Unresolved problems can lead to other serious problems with family, schools, and the criminal justice system. Much of the interest in identifying children's mental health problems has as its focus the understanding and prevention of disorders so as to reduce the risk of future difficulties.

Children's Mental Health Services

Interventions to treat children's mental health problems are based on a variety of theories about human development and behavior. Therapies used with children include those which are psychodynamically based, behaviorally based, and cognitively based, as well as those involving psychoactive medications.

Within the mental health system, a wide range of settings has been developed to treat children's mental health problems. These settings —from psychiatric hospitals to outpatient mental health clinics—can be described as forming a continuum of intensiveness. Mental health authorities agree that it is desirable to provide treatment in the "least restrictive setting" possible. Severely disturbed children sometimes need intensive and restrictive service settings such as hospitals or RTCs. Typically, however, intensive settings such as these are needed only for relatively brief periods, with followup care in less restrictive environments such as community-based outpatient programs.

The choice of treatment and treatment setting for each mentally disturbed child is based on several factors. Certainly, the symptoms and the severity of the child's disorder are primary. Other factors that play a part in treatment decisions include the child's developmental status, the availability of family support, social and environmental conditions, the availability of financing for services, and the geographic availability of certain services.

Opportunities for preventing and treating children's mental health problems arise not only in the mental health system but within the educational, health care, child welfare, and juvenile justice systems. Models for providing mental health services in these settings have been developed. Programs to integrate mental health and other services at Federal, State, and local levels have also been developed. Such programs include individual case manager programs, with professionals to advocate for necessary and comprehensive treatment and to represent the child before all relevant programs so that services are coordinated.

Effectiveness of Mental Health Treatment and Preventive Services

Clinical and policy decisions based on knowledge about the effectiveness and appropriateness of services, rather than on their availability, would be desirable, but drawing firm conclusions about the effectiveness of treatment, treatment settings, and preventive services for children's mental health problems is difficult. The research base is limited and not methodologically rigorous.

Overall, however, OTA's analysis indicates that treatment is better than no treatment and that there is substantial evidence for the effectiveness of many specific treatments. Behavioral treatment, for example, is clearly effective for phobias and enuresis, and cognitive-behavioral therapy is effective for a range of disorders involving self-control (except aggressive behavior). Group therapy has been found to be effective with delinquent adolescents, and family therapy appears to be effective for children with conduct disorders and psychophysiological disorders. Psychopharmacological treatment, while not curative, has been found to have limited effectiveness with children with attention deficit disorder and hyperactivity (ADD-H), depression, or enuresis, and also in managing the behavior of children who are severely disturbed. Further, more rigorous research may demonstrate the usefulness of several other treatments for which there is preliminary evidence of effectiveness.

Questions about the effectiveness of mental health treatment in psychiatric hospitals and RTCs are difficult to answer because of the lack of systematic research. The lack of methodologically sound evidence for the effectiveness of mental health treatment provided through psychiatric hospitals and RTCs does not necessarily imply that these treatment settings are inappropriate—only that there is no solid evidence one way or the other. Whether or not some mentally disturbed children would be better off in alternative treatment settings is not known.

Available research on treatment settings does offer some evidence to support the potential effectiveness of a system of services ranging from outpatient community-based care to intensive residential-based care. The long-term effectiveness of psychiatric hospitalization and other forms of residential treatment, for example, appears to be related to the presence and quality of followup care. The effectiveness of day or night hospitalization appears to be related to the inclusion of the family in treatment plans.

Additional information about treatment effectiveness could be used to revise financial incen-

tives—both public and private—to promote the delivery of mental health care in the least restrictive setting possible for effective treatment, while permitting reimbursement for the range of services necessary. Thus, a more comprehensive and appropriate mental health treatment delivery system could be developed.

The effectiveness of prevention programs, whether developed primarily as a mental health intervention or designed as part of other service systems such as schools, is supported by several studies. Interventions to provide family support, for example, appear to have substantial potential to prevent and remedy a range of mental health problems and lead to better school achievement in children. Prevention programs in schools and preschools and pregnancy prevention programs for teenagers have also been found to be effective. Not only have many prevention programs led to positive changes in social, emotional, and academic measures, but such programs appear capable of preventing later governmental expenditures through the justice and welfare systems.

The important questions, rather than being about the *overall* effectiveness of children's mental health services, may be:

- what specific types of services are effective?
- under what conditions?
- for which children?
- at what developmental level?
- with which problems?
- under what environmental and family conditions?
- in what settings? and
- with what followup or concomitant parental, family, school, and other systems interventions?

Current Federal Efforts

State governments play the major role in providing and financing children's mental health services, although Federal Government and private sector roles are substantial. The Federal Government finances treatment for children's mental disorders primarily through the Alcohol, Drug Abuse, and Mental Health block grant, the Medicaid program, and the Civilian Health and Medical Program of the Uniformed Services. These and other financing programs also influence financing policy in the private sector.

Federal involvement in health, welfare, nutrition, and social services for children is also considerable; and Federal programs in these areas probably have a major impact in preventing and alleviating mental health problems, although their actual impact is difficult to measure. However, the lack of cohesive policies toward children, and across service programs, may create difficulties for those who would move public policy toward the continuum of care that many observers conclude is needed to address children's mental health needs.

Past national studies have observed that few mental health policies and programs—public or private—appear to take into account the complexity of influences in children's lives. Fragmentation of treatment programs and support services has resulted. Currently, programs at the Federal, State, and local levels are attempting to promote integration of services across professional, agency, and geographic boundaries. The Federal Child and Adolescent Service System Program, for example, provides grants to States to improve coordination among service systems, thus improving access to appropriate mental health services. The State Comprehensive Mental Health Services Plan Act of 1986 will institute another grant program to assist States to develop comprehensive services for the chronically mentally ill of all ages.

The Federal Government is virtually the only source of training and research support in the mental health area. Despite Federal programs of student assistance, the number of trained professionals available to deliver children's mental health services remains far below all estimates of the need. Currently, about 15 percent of NIMH's training funds appears to be directed to training clinicians to treat children.

A major difficulty in development of this background paper and in designing more effective children's mental health programs was the lack of data on many treatment regimens and service systems. Although NIMH commits approximately 20 percent of its current research budget to children's issues, available dollars have not kept pace with

assessments of the funds necessary. Most mental health care interventions are appropriate for evaluation studies—and most could benefit from the information that research provides. In addition, basic information about the characteristics and utilization of the contemporary mental health service system is not available. The financial savings from a more comprehensive database are potentially enormous; the benefits to children and society of more effective programs are incalculable.

Conclusion

OTA's analysis suggests several needs in relation to children's mental health problems and services. Two needs are: a more informed estimate of the number of children who require mental health services, and a description of the availability and use of children's mental health services.

A more immediate need is for improved delivery of mental health services to children. Clearly, the mental health services currently available to children are inadequate, despite a substantial theoretical and research base suggesting that mental health interventions for children are effective.

The need for improved children's mental health services is not new; it has been highlighted by a number of past national studies and commissions. If the need is to be met, changes may be necessary in the way mental health services are conceptualized, financed, and provided. In an ideal system, an adequate range and number of preventive, treatment, and aftercare services would be available, particularly in the communities where children reside, so that families and others can be involved. Access to treatment on an outpatient basis, and before a child develops a diagnosable disorder, seems especially important. Access to treatment could be facilitated by reducing restrictions on mental health benefits.

OTA found that new efforts to coordinate services between the mental health system and other systems that children may come in contact with— the general health care, educational, social welfare, and juvenile justice systems—are encouraging to many mental health professionals. These new coordination programs may result in new efforts to detect and treat mental health problems.

Finally, additional information about the causes of mental health problems, the services available to prevent and treat them, the extent to which the services are used, and the effectiveness of a variety of promising approaches could greatly aid the development of a system that would match the mental health needs of children.

Part I: Earlier Evaluations and the Current Situation

Earlier Evaluations and the Current Situation

Earlier Evaluations and the Current Situation

INTRODUCTION

Services for children[1] with mental health problems have long been a focus of national concern. This chapter summarizes the work of several major policy-related studies and commissions, giving

___
[1]Throughout this background paper, the term "children" is used to refer generally to all infants, children, and adolescents under age 18. Where necessary, further distinctions are drawn among children of various ages and developmental stages.

their conclusions about the prevalence of mental health problems in children and their recommendations for services. The chapter also presents available information pertaining to trends in the availability and use of children's mental health services. Although data to assess the current situation are limited, it is nevertheless clear that several key policy recommendations of past studies and commissions have yet to be implemented.

EARLIER EVALUATIONS OF CHILDREN'S MENTAL HEALTH NEEDS AND SERVICES

Estimates of the Prevalence of Children's Mental Health Problems

Estimating the prevalence of mental health problems among children is hard for several reasons. Distinguishing between distinct mental health problems and normal changes during a child's development, for example, is often difficult. Also, some children without a diagnosable disorder may require mental health services because of problems in their social and physical environment (see ch. 4). These factors complicate the task of enumerating specific disorders and identifying children in need.

To complicate matters further, various panels that have tried to estimate the prevalence of children's mental health problems in the past have varied in the age range of children and the types of problems included in their estimates. Also, because of changes in psychiatric nomenclature, prevalence estimates used in individual studies or reports cannot be reliably replicated by subsequent groups. Nevertheless, all of the various panels' estimates have been roughly similar (see table 1), and the panels have all agreed that the need for children's mental health services exceeds the availability of services.

Joint Commission on the Mental Health of Children (1969)

One of the most detailed assessments of the magnitude of children's mental health problems was conducted by the Joint Commission on the Mental Health of Children (324). Established in 1965 (Public Law 89-97), the Joint Commission on the Mental Health of Children was specifically mandated to develop a coordinated study of the diagnosis, prevention, and treatment of "emotional illness" in children and adolescents. An earlier commission whose work had led to the 1963 act establishing community mental health centers throughout the country had not dealt explicitly with children (324).

In defining and estimating the prevalence of emotional disorders in children, the Joint Commission was hindered by a lack of specific diagnostic criteria. The Joint Commission adopted a rather broad definition of an "emotionally disturbed child" based on its synthesis of research and expert opinion:

. . . one who'se progressive personality development is interfered with or arrested by a variety of factors, so that he shows an impairment in the capacity expected of him for his age and endow-

Table 1.—Estimates of Children With Mental Health Needs[a]

	Children under 18 years of age with mental health needs	
	Percent	Number[b]
All mentally disturbed children:		
Joint Commission on the Mental Health of Children (1969)	13.6%	8.8 million
President's Commission on Mental Health (1978)	5% to 15%	3.0 to 9.6 million
Gould, et al. (1981)	11.8%[c]	7.5 million
Severely mentally disturbed children:		
National Plan for the Chronically Mentally Ill (1980)	8%	9.1 million
Knitzer/CDF (1982)	5.0%	3 million

[a]Estimates differ because inconsistent definitions of children's mental health needs have been used. The U.S. Department of Health and Human Services is currently evaluating the validity of a diagnostic interview schedule for use with children in order to conduct an epidemiological study of the presence of mental disorders.
[b]The number of children in need of services is calculated as a percent of the 1980 population of 63.8 million individuals under 18 years of age.
[c]Subsequent analyses concur with this estimate. See text.

SOURCES: Joint Commission on the Mental Health of Children, *Crisis in Child Mental Health: Challenge for the 1970's* (New York: Harper & Row, 1969); President's Commission on Mental Health, *Report to the President From the President's Commission on Mental Health*, vol. 1 (Commission Report) and vol. 3 (Task Panel Reports) (Washington, DC: U.S. Government Printing Office, 1978); M.S. Gould, R. Wunsch-Hitzig, and B. Dohrenwend, "Estimating the Prevalence of Childhood Psychopathology: A Critical Review," *Journal of the American Academy of Child Psychiatry* 20:462, 1981; L. Silver, "Chronic Mental Illness in Children and Adolescents: Scope of the Problem," paper for the National Conference on Chronic Mental Illness in Children and Adolescents, sponsored by the American Psychiatric Association, Dallas, TX, March 1985. J. Knitzer, *Unclaimed Children* (Washington, DC: Children's Defense Fund, 1982).

ment; (1) for reasonably accurate perception of the world around him; (2) for impulse control; (3) for satisfying and satisfactory relations with others; (4) for learning; or (5) for any combination of these.

Using this definition to interpret available research, the Joint Commission on the Mental Health of Children estimated that up to 13.6 percent of children were "emotionally disturbed." This included a small percentage (0.6 percent) of children who were considered psychotic, 2 to 3 percent who were severely disturbed, and an additional 8 to 10 percent who suffered from emotional problems serious enough to require mental health services.

U.S. Department of Health, Education, and Welfare: Project on the Classification of Exceptional Children (1975)

The issues of classifying children's mental health problems were also of concern subsequent to the Joint Commission's report. In 1972, a project was initiated by the Secretary of the U.S. Department of Health, Education, and Welfare (DHEW), now the U.S. Department of Health and Human Services, to consider issues in the classification of "exceptional" children, including but not limited to those with mental health problems. Supported by a consortium of DHEW agencies and directed by Hobbs, the Project on the Classification of Exceptional Children brought together a group of experts to develop a better understanding of the issues involved in classification and a rationale for policy and services for "exceptional" children.

The final report of the project cited a DHEW Bureau of Education (298,299) estimate that there were about 7 million children aged 0 to 19 in various "exceptional" categories (physically handicapped, retarded, and emotionally disturbed), but it did not estimate prevalence for specific disabilities. Another 1 million children (2.9 percent of children aged 10 to 17) had been in trouble with the law in 1972, and 10 million poor and 10 million nonwhite children were also of concern to the advisors to DHEW.

The report concluded that although there were significant problems associated with labeling children, categorization was often necessary to establish policy and to ensure that services were delivered. The report noted, however, that the classification of emotional disorders was particularly difficult and therefore recommended the development of multidimensional classification systems. A central feature of this recommendation was that such systems classify disorders, rather than children.

President's Commission on Mental Health and Its Task Panel on Infants, Children, and Adolescents (1978)

The President's Commission on Mental Health was established in 1977 to undertake a broadbased review of national mental health needs and to make recommendations to the President as to how those needs might be met (514). One of the principal "task panels" of the Commission addressed the mental health needs of children. Using studies conducted since the time of the Joint Commission on the Mental Health of Children, this task panel estimated that from 5 to 15 percent of children aged 3 to 15 had handicapping mental health problems. The panel's lower estimate corresponds to estimates of the number of psychotic and severely disturbed children; its higher estimate corresponds to the number of children with "neuroses" and behavior problems for whom mental health intervention may be useful.

The Commission as a whole stated that the country's mental health problems could not "be defined only in terms of disabling mental illnesses and identified psychiatric disorders." Mental health problems "must include the damage to mental health associated with unrelenting poverty and unemployment and the institutionalized discrimination that occurs on the basis of race, sex, class, age, and mental or physical handicaps," and "conditions that involve emotional or psychological distress which do not fit conventional categories of classification or services" (514).

Recent Estimates of the Prevalence of Children's Mental Health Problems

Epidemiologic research on mental health problems needed in order to estimate prevalence has continued to develop. Over two dozen studies of the prevalence of mental disorders in children and adolescents have now been conducted (229,248, 389,609).

Some of the most important research on prevalence, conducted in the United Kingdom by Rutter and colleagues (562,566), is believed to be relevant to the situation in the United States. On the basis of a convergence of identifications by mental health professionals, parents, and teachers, Rutter estimated that 13.2 percent of children in the United Kingdom were in need of mental health services.

In a detailed 1981 review, Gould, et al., concluded that the percentage of children and adolescents in need of mental health services in the United States was probably "no lower than 11.8 percent" (248). Later reviews, by Gilmore, et al. (229), and Silver (609), concur with the 11.8-percent figure.

Gould and her colleagues' estimate that about 12 percent of the children in the United States—7.5 million—are in need of mental health services seems to be one on which there is general concurrence. This estimate, however, reveals nothing about the severity of disturbances and levels

of care children need—distinctions that are essential for the development of comprehensive public policy.

Increasing interest is being directed to children with severe mental health disturbances, both in terms of identification and for developing appropriate treatment options (396). Estimates of the number of severely disturbed children, however, differ substantially. In comparison to the findings of the President's Commission on Mental Health (514), for example, the 1980 National Plan for the Chronically Mentally Ill (609) estimated that about 9.1 million (8 percent) children are severely disturbed and in need of services.

Recommendations About Mental Health Services for Children

Concern about the inadequacy of mental health services for children is not a recent phenomenon. As long ago as 1909, a White House Conference on Children recommended new programs to care for mentally disturbed children (324). A White House Conference in 1930 echoed the earlier recommendation and maintained that mentally disturbed children have the "right" to develop the way other children do. A similar conclusion has been reached by nearly every subsequent commission or panel (324). These panels and study commissions have made numerous detailed and specific recommendations conceiving policy relevant to the mental health needs of children. Only the flavor of their recommendations can be provided here. Selected conclusions and recommendations of various commissions and panels are summarized in table 2, and the work of the more recent groups is discussed in detail below.

Joint Commission on the Mental Health of Children (1969)

The Joint Commission on the Mental Health of Children (324), in its 1969 report *Crisis in Child Mental Health*, stated that large numbers of emotionally, physically, and socially handicapped children did not receive necessary or appropriate services and that the mental health service system for children and youth was wholly inadequate. Although the most disturbed and disrup-

Table 2.—Mental Health Services for Children: Selected Findings and Recommendations of Past National Study Panels

Selected conclusions	Selected recommendations	Subsequent Federal actions
White House Conference on Children (1909):		
	Develop new programs to care for emotionally disturbed children.	
White House Conference on Children (1930):		
Emotionally disturbed children have the ''right'' to develop like other children.	Develop new programs to care for emotionally disturbed children.	
Joint Commission on the Mental Health of Children (1969):		
Large numbers of emotionally, physically, and socially handicapped children do not receive necessary or appropriate services.	Establish a child advocacy system to coordinate Federal, State, and local action. Establish community services focused on prevention and remediation. Expand prevention services to include family planning, prenatal care, nutrition, and other physical health care. Deliver treatment in settings resembling normal living conditions Increase research on diagnosis and treatment.	
Project on the Classification of Exceptional Children (1975):		
Services for all kinds of children remain a tangled thicket of conceptual confusions, competing authorities, contrary purposes, and professional rivalries, leading to the fragmentation of services and the lack of sustained attention to the needs of individual children and their families.	Classify disorders, not children. Coordinate and plan services. Educate all children; make public schools advocates for all services for all children.	Education for All Handicapped Children Act (Public Law 94-142) passed in 1975.
President's Commission on Mental Health or its Task Panel on Infants, Children, and Adolescents (1978):		
A delay in the delivery of mental health services is no more justifiable than a delay in the delivery of physical health services. Adolescents are one of the most underserved groups in Nation. Mental health commissions have to date garnered little action for minority group programs.	Provide prevention services (e.g., prenatal care) to all families with children. Services should ''respect ethnic differences,'' be adapted to children's specific needs, treat significant others. Incorporate mental health services (e.g., developmental assessments, diagnostic services) into general health care. Involve parents in development of treatment, educational, and service plans. Develop a network of psychiatric, pediatric, counseling, special education, and occupational training services. Organize mental health services along a continuum of intensiveness. Increase residential and outpatient care. Make mental health care available at reasonable costs to all who need it. Address adolescent suicide, teenage pregnancy, delinquency, and substance abuse. Increase the number of mental health professionals trained to work with children. Fund more basic and evaluation research.	Mental Health Systems Act (1980) authorized programs to improve the delivery and coordination of services for severely emotionally disturbed children and adolescents (repealed in 1981).
Select Panel for the Promotion of Child Health (1981):		
Public Law 94-142 (the Education for All Handicapped Children Act) has wrought significant improvements, but substantial variations exist in the availability of services.	Develop better means of identifying and evaluating children with handicapping conditions, including serious emotional disturbance. Require delivery of health and mental health services to handicapped children. Improve Federal and State monitoring, technical assistance, and enforcement of Public Law 94-142. Expand mental health services to include early detection and treatment of developmental problems, other preventive services for children and families, high quality residential treatment services, and community support mechanisms. Develop new means of coordinating physical and mental health services, and mental health services with educational and social services. Involve families in delivery of mental health services.	
Knuitzer/Children's Defense Fund Survey of State Mental Health Programs:		
All services (residential and nonresidential) are inadequate. Inpatient psychiatric care is the most accessible, but also the most costly and restrictive. States do not monitor children's progression through mental health system. Service systems (juvenile, educational, child welfare, mental health) are uncoordinated. Seriously emotionally disturbed children appear to be underserved under Public Law 94-142.	Increase efforts to identify children and adolescents in need of services or who are inappropriately served. Develop incentives for creating coordinated services. Coordinate juvenile justice, education, child welfare, and mental health services by means of a child advocacy system. Target Federal Alcohol, Drug Abuse & Mental Health (ADM) block grant funds for children's services.	Child and Adolescent Service System Program (CASSP) was funded to promote coordination of mental health services within States. Ten percent of ADM mental health block grant funds was set aside for children or other underserved populations.

SOURCES: Joint Commission on the Mental Health of Children, *Crisis in Child Mental Health: Challenge for the 1970's* (New York: Harper & Row, 1969); N. Hubbs, *The Futures of Children: Categories, Labels and Their Consequences* (San Francisco, CA: Jossey-Bass, 1975); President's Commission on Mental Health, *Report to the President From the President's Commission on Mental Health*, vol. 1 (Commission Report) and vol. 3 (Task Panel Reports) (Washington, DC: U.S. Government Printing Office, 1978); Select Panel for the Promotion of Child Health, *Better Health for Our Children: A National Strategy*, presented to the U.S. Congress and the Secretary of Health and Human Services, Washington, DC, 1981; J. Knitzer, *Unclaimed Children* (Washington, DC: Children's Defense Fund, 1982).

tive children could receive treatment services, the Commission found that treatment provided to them very often was inappropriate and ineffective. The Joint Commission was particularly concerned that severely disturbed children were being institutionalized in State mental hospitals and that such facilities provided custodial rather than treatment services for children. The Joint Commission was also concerned about the "corrosive" effects of poverty and the fact that mental health problems were more acute and services less available among poor children.

A principal recommendation of the Joint Commission on the Mental Health of Children was that a child advocacy system be established to coordinate Federal, State, and local actions. The Commission believed that advocacy was essential for development of a comprehensive network to meet children's mental health, physical, and social needs.

The Joint Commission also recommended the establishment of community services that focused on prevention and "remediation." Recommended prevention services included family planning, prenatal care, and mental health services associated with schools. Remedial mental health services, which the Commission estimated would be required for 10 percent of children, were to be based on children's functional level, rather than on legal or clinical classification systems.

The Joint Commission further recommended that children (particularly the severely handicapped) be cared for in settings that most closely resembled normal living situations. An additional recommendation was for increased research on diagnosis and treatment of children's mental health problems. The Joint Commission believed that both basic and applied research was essential and suggested a variety of research priorities, both for the National Institute of Mental Health (NIMH) and for the National Institutes of Health.

U.S. Department of Health, Education, and Welfare: Project on the Classification of Exceptional Children

Perhaps because it was concerned with "exceptional" children of several kinds (handicapped, disadvantaged, and delinquent), the Project on the Classification of Exceptional Children was per-

haps even more concerned than the Joint Commission on the Mental Health of Children with the coordination of services across agencies and categories of children. Thus, the Project's final report (298,299) recommended that the U.S. Congress and the legislative bodies of each State and community establish an agency to serve a planning and coordinating function for all programs bearing on families and children. The Project report also suggested that at every level, citizens' councils advise the planning agencies on program development and agency operations. The Project also made recommendations concerning specific programs which might be implemented under the purview of the legislative bodies, and noted several needs that should be given priority attention:

- support for parents,
- improved residential programs for children,
- fairness to disadvantaged and minority group children,
- improved classification systems,
- better organization of services, and
- new knowledge to inform policy.

One of the Project's recommendations, that all children including the handicapped have access to education, was implemented with the passage of Public Law 94-142, the Education for All Handicapped Children Act. Public Law 94-142 also implicitly made the public schools the primary

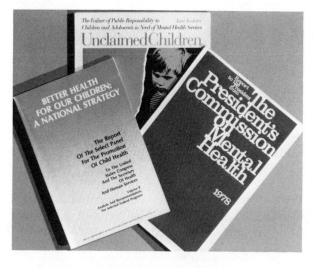

A number of national studies and commissions have concluded that mental health services for children are inadequate.

source of advocacy for children, another recommendation of the Project on the Classification of Exceptional Children.

President's Commission on Mental Health and Its Task Panel on Infants, Children, and Adolescents (1978)

The President's Commission on Mental Health (514) found that many of the Joint Commission's 1969 recommendations had not been implemented. Children and adolescents, the President's Commision found, continued to receive inadequate mental health care:

> Services that reflect the unique needs of children and adolescents are frequently unavailable. Our existing mental health services system contains too few mental health professionals and other personnel trained to meet the special needs of children and adolescents. Even when identified, children's needs are too often isolated into distinct categories, each to be addressed separately by a different specialist. Shuttling children from service to service, each with its own label, adds to their confusion, increases their despair, and sets the pattern for adult disability.

The Commission's subtask panel on infants, children, and adolescents recommended preventive services for all children, not only those identified as mentally disturbed. Services such as developmental assessments and access to diagnostic mental health services, it suggested, should be incorporated within children's general health care.

The subtask panel also recommended a network of "psychiatric, pediatric, counseling, special education and occupational training services" for children with severe psychiatric disorders. These services were necessary, according to the panel, because no matter how successful prevention efforts were, some children would always require special help. The services provided, the panel recommended, should be adapted to children's specific needs and should include counseling with parents and others significant in a child's life. In addition, the panel believed, it was essential that services "respect ethnic differences."

The subtask panel on infants, children, and adolescents emphasized that children's mental health services should be provided within a system of care that "insofar as possible maintain a continuing relationship between child and family." To prevent disruption in the relationship between children and their families, the panel recommended that health insurance plans eliminate barriers to reimbursement for outpatient treatment services. The panel also recommended that parents be involved in the development of special education and other treatment plans, especially for intensive services provided for severely disturbed children.

Another recommendation of the subtask panel was that children's mental health services be organized along a continuum of intensiveness, so that children could move along the continuum as their needs changed. Good residential facilities specializing in the treatment of severely disturbed children and adolescents, the panel suggested, were urgently needed. The panel supported the Joint Commission calling for development of a better research and evaluation base, characterizing the tendency to reduce research funding in order to provide treatment services as "penny wise and pound foolish" (514). Noting that without more research and evaluation, "the potential for waste of resources is great," the panel recommended a 10-percent set-aside of total program funds for research, demonstrations, and evaluation.

The subtask panel called the mental health system for adolescents "woefully inadequate," noting that adolescents were one of the most underserved groups in the Nation. This panel urged that services be provided to address such problems as adolescent suicide, teenage pregnancy, delinquency, and substance abuse. The panel's recommendations focused on development of an integrated network of mental health services in schools, juvenile courts, neighborhood centers, and occupational training facilities.

One impact of the work of the President's Commission was the development and enactment of the Mental Health Systems Act. The act authorized programs to improve the delivery and coordination of services for severely emotionally disturbed children and adolescents. The act became law in 1981, but was repealed before it became effective and was replaced by the Alcohol, Drug Abuse, and Mental Health (ADM) block grant (Public Law 97-35; see ch. 10).

Select Panel for the Promotion of Child Health (1981)

Established at about the same time as the President's Commission on Mental Health was the Select Panel for the Promotion of Child Health established under Public Law 95-626. The Select Panel had a broad mandate; it attempted to develop recommendations that:

> . . . reflect[ed] hardheaded analysis of serious unmet needs in child and maternal health . . . and a sober and pragmatic assessment of the capacity of our institutions to provide parents, professionals and . . . others working to improve child health with the scientific, financial and organizational support they need.

The Select Panel reported its findings in December 1980 (595). The general recommendations of the Panel, much like those of its predecessors, emphasized the interrelationships among services provided by health care agencies, schools, families, and social service institutions. The Select Panel's analysis suggested changes to a wide range of Federal programs affecting children. With respect to mental health needs, the Panel focused on implementation of the Education for All Handicapped Children Act (Public Law 94-142, enacted in 1975) and mental health service systems that were to be affected by the Mental Health Systems Act (enacted in 1980, but then repealed in 1981).

Public Law 94-142 mandates that handicapped children be provided access to a free and appropriate public education. Public Law 94-142 authorizes a program for States to receive Federal funds, but it also "guarantees" the right to education for handicapped children without regard to the provision of Federal funds to support such services. Although the Select Panel found that significant improvements had resulted from Public Law 94-142, particularly in changing attitudes about the handicapped, it was concerned that substantial variations existed across States in the availability of services. The Panel stressed the need for better methods of identifying and evaluating children with handicapping conditions and more stringent requirements for delivering health and mental health services to these children. To ensure compliance with the law, it recommended Federal and State monitoring, technical assistance, and enforcement.

The Select Panel also considered the role of community mental health centers and other mental health service systems and recommended that these systems expand mental health services for children. Although children's mental health services had been mandated earlier (Part F of the 1970 Amendments to the Community Mental Health Centers Act), direct Federal support specifically for children's programs had been withdrawn in 1975. The Select Panel believed that developmental assessment and other preventive services, as well as high-quality residential treatment services and community support mechanisms, were necessary components of all comprehensive mental health programs.

As had the President's Commission on Mental Health in 1978, the Select Panel for the Promotion of Child Health recommended that mental health services be coordinated with general health care. The Select Panel also recommended coordination of education and social welfare programs that serve children. Other recommendations of the Select Panel were that community mental health programs provide services in schools, Head Start programs, and juvenile justice institutions, and that families be involved in the delivery of mental health services.

Knitzer/Children's Defense Fund (1982)

Concern about the adequacy of services for mentally disturbed children remained, despite the convergence of recommendations by the Joint Commission, the President's Commission, and the Select Panel. In 1982, the Children's Defense Fund (CDF) published an elaborate and highly critical study of how children and adolescents in need of mental health services are treated (358). That report, *Unclaimed Children*, by Jane Knitzer, described a survey of mental health services for severely disturbed children and adolescents in 50 States and the District of Columbia. Unlike the reports of earlier commissions and panels, the Knitzer/CDF report is based on systematically collected original data and is one of only a few efforts to comprehensively assess State, as well as Federal, programs.

The Knitzer/CDF report concluded that there were 3 million seriously disturbed children (based on the estimate of the President's Commission on

Mental Health in 1978), but that 2 million (two-thirds) of these children were not receiving needed treatment services. The report also suggested that many children who received services received inappropriate care and that poor and minority group children were most likely to receive no care or inappropriate care.

Using data from State and county hospitals, Knitzer concluded that the most restrictive and costly level of care—inpatient hospital treatment—was also the most accessible. Although the data Knitzer collected suggested that as many as 40 percent of such hospital placements were unsuitable, alternatives to hospital services for severely disturbed children were found to be either nonexistent or rudimentary in many States. One-third of the States responding to Knitzer's survey indicated a need for more long- or short-term beds. According to Knitzer (358):

> . . . those States with the fewest alternatives to inpatient care were generally the ones that wanted more beds. Those with a number of alternative

programs saw less need to fund more hospital placements . . .

Knitzer suggested that Federal funds had been used disproportionately to provide medically oriented inpatient care, while Federal resources available for community services had declined.

Responsibility for seriously disturbed children, according to Knitzer, lies with public agencies. The Knitzer/CDF report strongly recommended increased efforts to identify children and adolescents who are either in need of services or are being inappropriately served. It also urged the development of incentives to create a coordinated set of services appropriate to the child. As did the reports of each of the government panels described earlier, the Knitzer/CDF report recommended increased coordination among agencies that deal with children, including educational, juvenile justice, and child welfare agencies. A specific recommendation of the report was that ADM block grant funds be targeted for children's services.

THE CURRENT AVAILABILITY AND USE OF CHILDREN'S MENTAL HEALTH SERVICES

Despite general agreement among experts about the magnitude of children's mental health problems, it is difficult to specify precisely the number of children with mental health problems and the types of services they need. The National Institute of Mental Health (NIMH), which recently conducted a nationwide study of the prevalence of adult mental health disorders (533), plans a parallel survey of children's problems. At the time this background paper was being written, NIMH was studying the reliability and validity of the instrument it plans to use in the survey—the Diagnostic Interview Schedule for Children (DISC). DISC is based on the American Psychiatric Association's *Diagnostic and Statistical Manual of Mental Disorders*. The NIMH survey represents an important step toward more precise assessment of children's mental health problems (664).

A serious problem in attempting to assess the extent to which mental health services for children are available, and the degree to which the mental health service system has changed in re-

cent years, is the lack of precise epidemiologic data. The information available at the time this background paper was being prepared was quite dated. The most recent systematically collected information on inpatient, residential, and outpatient mental health care pertained to utilization for 1981 (665). These data do not reflect the impact of recent policy changes such as Medicare's Part A prospective payment system, the limitation by the Civilian Health and Medical Program of the Uniformed Services on inpatient treatment, the 10-percent set-aside in the mental health portion of the ADM block grant, and the Child and Adolescent Service System Program (see ch. 10). Nevertheless, they do allow the identification of several noteworthy trends. For the most part, the continuation of these trends has been confirmed by individuals consulted during the preparation of this background paper.

The most dramatic trend in recent years has been a decline in the number of children treated as inpatients in State and county mental hospitals (665). This trend has been accompanied, however, by increases in children's admissions to private psychiatric hospitals and to facilities such as psychiatric units of general hospitals, for a small net increase in children's admissions to psychiatric hospitals.

In 1970, as shown in table 3, the rate of children's admissions to private psychiatric hospitals (9.3 per 100,000 children under 18) was one-fourth the rate of children's admissions to State and county mental hospitals (37.8 per 100,000 children under 18). During the 1970s, children's admissions to State and county mental hospitals declined 30 percent and admissions to private psychiatric hospitals increased almost 200 percent, so that in 1980, the latest period for which systematic data are available, the rates of children's admissions were about the same for both types of institutions. The rates of children's admissions to non-Federal general hospitals with inpatient psychiatric services increased slightly from 63.3 per 100,000 population in 1970 to 68.5 per 100,000 population in 1980, for a total net increase in the rate of psychiatric hospitalization of children of about 10 admissions per 100,000 population. There may be significant regional variations (589).

Some evidence suggests that the length of treatment episodes in State and county mental hospitals is declining, although the evidence on the length of stay for children in private psychiatric hospitals is unclear (458,665). As can be seen in table 4, data from NIMH indicate that the median length of stay of children in State and county mental hospitals dropped from 74 days in 1970 to 54 days in 1980, while the length of stay in private psychiatric hospitals remained constant at 36 days (665). A survey of National Association of Private Psychiatric Hospitals members, however, found that the median length of stay for children in 1985 in the private hospitals surveyed was twice NIMH's number for 1980 (458). Data from NIMH indicate that the length of stay in non-Federal general hospitals with inpatient psychiatric services increased from 9 to 17 days between 1970 and 1975, then decreased to 14 days in 1980. The evidence just cited clearly shows that general hospitals are used for short-term care, and the length of stay in State and county mental hospitals has declined. It does not allow conclusions about the length of treatment in private psychiatric hospitals.

As shown in table 3, NIMH data suggest that there has been an increase in utilization of residential treatment centers for emotionally disturbed children (RTCs). Such facilities can provide an alternative form of treatment for children who require residential treatment but who do not require constant medical supervision (see ch. 6). There was a substantial increase in the number of admissions to RTCs between 1969 and 1981. According to NIMH data, the rate more than doubled, from 11.4 admissions per 100,000 population under 18 in 1969 to 28.3 admissions per 100,000 pop-

Table 3.—Admissions of Children Under 18 Years of Age to Hospital Inpatient Psychiatric Facilities and Residential Treatment Centers, 1970, 1975, and 1980[a]

	1970[b]		1975		1980[c]	
	Rate[d]	Number	Rate[d]	Number	Rate[d]	Number
Hospital inpatient facilities						
State and county mental hospitals[e]	37.8	26,352	38.1	25,252	26.1	16,612
Private psychiatric hospitals............................	9.3	6,452	23.3	15,426	26.3	16,735
Non-Federal general hospitals with inpatient psychiatric services	63.3	44,135	64.4	42,690	68.5	43,595
Total hospital inpatient admissions	110.4	76,939	125.8	83,368	120.9	76,942
Residential treatment centers for emotionally disturbed children (RTCs)	11.4	7,596	18.8	12,022	28.3	17,703

[a]Includes new admissions and readmissions during the year, so is not an unduplicated count.
[b]Data for RTCs are for 1969.
[c]Data for RTCs are for 1981.
[d]Rate per 100,000 children under 18 years of age.
[e]Includes St. Elizabeth's Hospital in Washington, DC.

SOURCE: National Institute of Mental Health, Alcohol, Drug Abuse, and Mental Health Administration, Public Health Service, U.S. Department of Health and Human Services, *Mental Health, United States, 1985*, C.A. Taube and S.A. Barrett (eds.), DHHS Pub. No. (ADM) 85-1378 (Rockville, MD: 1985), tables 2.21 and 2.3.

Table 4.—Median Length of Stay in Hospital Inpatient Psychiatric Facilities Among Children Under 18 Years of Age, 1970, 1975, and 1980

	1970	1975	1980
State and county mental hospitals	74 days	66 days	54 days
Private psychiatric hospitals	36 days	36 days	36 days
Non-Federal general hospitals with inpatient psychiatric services	9 days	17 days	14 days

SOURCE: National Institute of Mental Health, Alcohol, Drug Abuse, and Mental Health Administration, Public Health Service, U.S. Department of Health and Human Services, *Mental Health, United States, 1985,* C.A. Taube and S.A. Barrett (eds.), DHHS Pub. No. (ADM) 85-1378 (Rockville, MD: 1985).

ulation under 18 in 1981. The declining use of State and county mental hospitals and increasing use of RTCs is shown dramatically in figure 3.

Partial hospitalization or day treatment in other facilities is another increasingly accepted way to treat some children. It may be appropriate for those who require mental health care that is more intensive than outpatient care but less intensive than inpatient or RTC care (see ch. 6). Data on children's admissions for partial hospitalization comparable to the data on other settings are not available, but the increasing use of partial hospitalization can be inferred from NIMH's 1983 end-of-year census data. These data indicated that 20,000 individuals under 18 were receiving a planned program of mental health treatment services generally provided in visits of 3 or more hours to groups of patients/clients in various settings (665).

The use of outpatient treatment mental health services by children is difficult to determine. The 1980 National Medical Care Utilization and Expenditures Survey found that 3.2 percent of children under 18—and 4.3 percent of all age groups combined—had had a mental health visit in 1980, (665). Some observers have suggested that these figures probably underestimate the number of individuals who receive outpatient mental health treatment and that the treatment rate for individuals of all ages may be as high as 6 percent (178). The 1980-82 NIMH epidemiologic catchment area survey of adults in urban areas found that 6 to 7 percent of those surveyed had had a visit for

Figure 3.—Admission Rates for Children Under 18 Years to Psychiatric Hospitals and Residential Treatment Centers, 1970, 1975, and 1980[a]

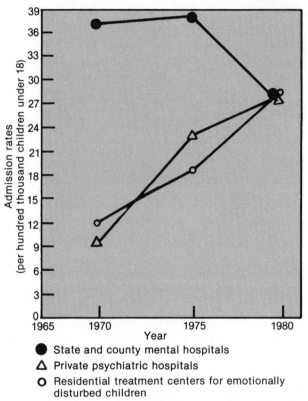

- ● State and county mental hospitals
- △ Private psychiatric hospitals
- ○ Residential treatment centers for emotionally disturbed children

[a]Data for residential treatment centers are for years 1969, 1975, and 1981.

SOURCES: **1970 to 1980 admission rates** to State and county mental hospitals and private psychiatric hospitals, and 1969, 1975, and 1981 admissions for residential treatment centers: National Institute of Mental Health, Alcohol, Drug Abuse and Mental Health Administration, Public Health Service, U.S. Department of Health and Human Services, *Mental Health United States, 1985,* C.A. Taube and S.A. Barrett (eds.), DHHS Pub. No. (ADM) 85-1378 (Rockville, MD: 1985). **1969, 1975 and 1980 population under 18** (used to calculate admission rates for residential treatment centers): U.S. Department of Commerce, Bureau of the Census, Washington, DC, unpublished data for 1969, 1975, and 1980.

a mental health problem, not necessarily a diagnosable disorder, in the 6-month period preceding the survey (599). Without specifying precise percentage increases by age, a 1985 NIMH report (665) noted that the use of outpatient mental health services had greatly increased for all ages. Careful assessment of the use of mental health services by children awaits conduct of the NIMH epidemiologic survey of children.

CONCLUSION

There appears to be a significant gap between the number of children identified in epidemiologic assessments as requiring mental health services and the number receiving services. There is general agreement that at least 12 percent of the Nation's children—7.5 million—are in need of some type of mental health treatment. Available evidence suggests that only a small number (fewer than one-third) of the children who have mental health problems receive treatment. An unknown number of other children may be at risk for mental health problems and in need of preventive services (see ch. 4). The problems of a lack of treatment and inappropriate treatment for children's mental health problems have long plagued those responsible for providing services to children. Subsequent chapters of this background paper examine the current state of knowledge about diagnosable mental disorders and the environmental risk factors that can cause or exacerbate children's mental health problems.

Part II: Problems

DSM-III Mental Disorders in Children

Chapter 3
DSM-III Mental Disorders in Children

INTRODUCTION

The mental health problems of children exist along a continuum. This chapter describes those problems which are considered mental *disorders* among children, as described in the most widely used diagnostic manual in the United States—the third edition of the American Psychiatric Association's *Diagnostic and Statistical Manual*, better known as "DSM-III"[1] (19). Generally, DSM-III defines a mental disorder as:

> . . . a clinically significant behavioral or psychological syndrome or pattern that occurs in an individual and that is typically associated with either a painful symptom (distress) or impairment in one or more areas of functioning (disability).

A description of the major DSM-III diagnosable disorders in children is important to an analysis of mental health services, because these disorders make up an intellectual framework by which the mental health professions understand children's mental health problems. It takes on added importance, because, in most cases, an individual must have a DSM-III diagnosable disorder to be eligible for third-party reimbursement for treatment.

For most mental health problems, the etiology is not known (19). However, many DSM-III disorders and other children's mental health problems are often related to environmental stressors such as poverty, parental divorce, and abuse and neglect. Environmental stressors that pose risks to children's mental health are described in chapter 4. Many observers believe that children exposed to such environmental stressors, in addition to children with diagnosable disorders, are in need of preventive or other mental health services discussed in this background paper. Both social and organic causes of mental disorders are continuously under investigation (668), but a comprehensive analysis of causation is beyond the scope of this background paper.

---

[1]At the time this background paper was being prepared, the American Psychiatric Association was revising DSM-III. The new version will be known as DSM-III-R.

THE DSM-III DIAGNOSTIC SYSTEM

A standard diagnostic system provides clinicians and researchers common terms with which to identify patients and thus makes possible sharing of information about similar classes of patients (19). It also allows clinicians and researchers to make use of experience with previous patients in planning and assessing the effectiveness of mental health treatment.

DSM-III provides clearer, more specific criteria for diagnoses than previous taxonomies have, and it bases the diagnoses on descriptive information about disorders rather than on causal factors, about which there is still disagreement. These aspects of DSM-III have been lauded, but criticisms of DSM-III have been raised as well (563). Some critics have objected to labeling children's mental health problems as "mental disorders" and have been concerned that DSM-III diagnoses would be used as labels to discriminate against children (563). Other criticisms are that DSM-III does not appropriately address mental health problems that do not fit into specific categories and lists specific criteria for diagnosis with little empirical basis for some categories (563).

DSM-III has gained substantial acceptance in the United States. Outside the United States, the ninth edition of the *International Classification of Diseases* (ICD-9), developed by the World Health Organization, is the standard.

DSM-III differs from ICD-9 and other classification systems in several respects. Among other things, it is the first widely used system to employ a multiaxial approach to the diagnostic evaluation of patients. The purpose of the multiaxial system of DSM-III is to "ensure that certain information that may be of value in planning treatment and predicting outcome for each individual is recorded" (19). DSM-III has five axes, each of which refers to a specific class of information relevant to a patient's mental health problems (see table 5).

The first three axes constitute the official diagnostic assessment. Axis I is for indicating all mental disorders other than those to be indicated on Axis II. Examples of Axis I disorders are anxiety disorder and major depression. Axis II is for longstanding personality disorders and specific disorders of development in which a child's development lags behind that of his or her peers in a specific area such as reading or arithmetic. A patient can receive multiple Axis I or Axis II diagnoses. Thus, for example, a child could be diagnosed as having an anxiety disorder (Axis I) in addition to a reading disorder (Axis II).

Axis III is used to note physical disorders or conditions that are relevant to understanding or managing a patient's mental health needs. The condition noted can be etiologically significant (e.g., a neurologic disorder associated with dementia) or not. This axis would be used, for example, to indicate juvenile diabetes, an illness that can have implications for the management of mental health care.

DSM-III explicitly recognizes that factors such as environmental stress and previous adaptation can influence the course and treatment of a mental health problem. A comprehensive DSM-III diagnosis includes information on these factors on Axes IV and V. Axis IV is a rating of the severity of any psychosocial stressors connected with the onset of a mental disorder. Examples of such stressors are shown in table 5.

Finally, Axis V is a rating of the patient's highest level of adaptive functioning, a composite of a patient's ability to manage social relations, occupation, and leisure time. Such information is often important in predicting the course of a disorder and in planning treatment (19).

In classifying mental disorders, DSM-III separates the class of disorders that usually first be-

Table 5.—DSM-III's Multiaxial Diagnostic Evaluation System

Official DSM-III Diagnostic Evaluation (Axes I, II, and III)

Mental Disorders [a,b]

Axis I: All Mental Disorders Not Assigned to Axis II
- Mental disorders not assigned to Axis II (e.g., depression, anxiety disorder, conduct disorder)
- Conditions not attributable to a mental disorder that are a focus of attention or treatment (e.g., academic problem, parent-child problem, isolated acts of child or adolescent antisocial behavior)
- Additional codes (e.g., unspecified mental disorder, no diagnosis on Axis I, no diagnosis on Axis II)

Axis II: Personality Disorders and Specific Developmental Disorders
- Personality disorders (e.g., paranoid personality disorder)[c]
- Specific developmental disorders (e.g., developmental reading disorder)

Physical Disorders and Conditions

Axis III: Physical Disorders and Conditions
- Any physical disorders or conditions that are potentially relevant to the understanding or management of the individual (e.g., diabetes in a child with conduct disorder)

Additional Information (Axes IV and V)

Axis IV: Severity of Psychosocial Stressors
- A rating on a scale of 1 (no apparent stressor) to 7 (catastrophic stressor) of the severity of the summed effect of all of the psychosocial stressors judged to have been a significant contributor to the development or exacerbation of the current disorder. Examples of psychosocial stressors that might be considered in the case of a child or adolescent include puberty, change in residence, overtly hostile relationship between parents, hostile parental behavior toward child, insufficient or inconsistent parental control, anomalous family situation (e.g., single parent, foster family), institutional rearing, school problems, legal problems, unwanted pregnancy, insufficient social or cognitive stimulation, natural or manmade disaster. A physical disorder can also be a psychosocial stressor if its impact is due to its meaning to the individual, in which case it would be noted on both Axis III and Axis IV.

Axis V: Highest Level of Adaptive Functioning Past Year
- A rating on a scale of 1 (superior) to 5 (poor) of an individual's highest level of adaptive functioning (for at least a few months) during the past year. Adaptive functioning is a composite of social relations, occupational/academic functioning, and use of leisure time.

[a]Mental disorders are disorders for which the manifestations are primarily behavioral or psychological; physical disorders are disorders for which the manifestations are not primarily behavioral or psychological.

[b]A person may have multiple diagnoses on Axes I and II—e.g., one diagnosis on Axis I and one diagnosis on Axis II, or multiple diagnoses within Axis I or Axis II.

[c]The diagnosis of a personality disorder is generally reserved for adults, although the manifestations of personality disorders may appear in childhood or adolescence.

SOURCE: Adapted from American Psychiatric Association, *Diagnostic and Statistical Manual of Mental Disorders*, 3d ed. (Washington, DC: 1980).

come evident in infants, children, or adolescents from several other major classes of disorders that are not generally restricted to children (see table 6). For heuristic purposes, DSM-III groups mental disorders that usually manifest themselves in

Table 6.—Children's Mental Disorders Listed in DSM-III[a]

MENTAL DISORDERS THAT ARE USUALLY FIRST EVIDENT IN INFANCY, CHILDHOOD, OR ADOLESCENCE

Intellectual Disorders

Mental retardation
   Mild mental retardation, moderate retardation, severe mental retardation, unspecified mental retardation

Developmental Disorders

Pervasive developmental disorders (PDDs)
   Infantile autism (onset before 30 months of age), childhood-onset pervasive developmental disorder (onset after 30 months of age and before 12 years of age)
Specific developmental disorders (SDDs) (Axis II of DSM-III)
   Developmental reading disorder (dyslexia), developmental arithmetic disorder, developmental language disorder (expressive type or receptive type), developmental articulation disorder, mixed specific developmental disorder, atypical specific developmental disorder

Behavior Disorders

Attention deficit disorder (ADD)
   ADD with hyperactivity, ADD without hyperactivity
Conduct disorder
   Undersocialized, aggressive; undersocialized, nonaggressive; socialized, aggressive; socialized, nonaggressive; atypical

Emotional Disorders

Anxiety disorders of childhood or adolescence
   Separation anxiety disorder; avoidant disorder of childhood or adolescence; overanxious disorder
Other disorders of infancy, childhood, or adolescence
   Reactive attachment disorder of infancy; schizoid disorder of childhood or adolescence; elective mutism; oppositional disorder; identity disorder

Physical (Psychophysiological) Disorders

Stereotyped movement disorders
   Transient tic disorder, chronic motor tic disorder, Tourette's disorder, atypical tic disorder, atypical stereotyped movement disorder
Eating disorders
   Anorexia nervosa, bulimia, pica
Other disorders with physical manifestations
   Stuttering, enuresis (repeated involuntary voiding of urine), encopresis (repeated voluntary or involuntary defecation in inappropriate places), sleepwalking disorder, sleep terror disorder

OTHER MENTAL DISORDERS THAT MAY AFFECT CHILDREN[b]

Organic mental disorders (e.g., delirium, dementia, alcohol intoxication, barbiturate intoxication)
Substance use disorders—sometimes occur in teens
   Abuse of or dependence on any of five classes of substances; alcohol, barbiturates, opioids, amphetamines, and cannabis
   Abuse of any of three classes of substances: cocaine, phencyclidine (PCP), and hallucinogens
   Dependence on tobacco
   Other, mixed, or unspecified substance abuse (e.g., glue sniffing)
   Dependence on a combination of substances (e.g., heroin and barbiturates, amphetamines and barbiturates)
Schizophrenic disorders (e.g., disorganized, catatonic, paranoid, or undifferentiated type)—onset is usually in late adolescence or early adulthood
Schizophreniform disorder
Affective disorders
   Major depression (single episode, recurrent)—can occur at any age, including infancy
Anxiety disorders
   Phobic disorders:
      Social phobia—often begins in late childhood or early adolescence
      Simple phobia (e.g., of animals, heights, school, water)—age at onset varies, but fear of animals almost always begins in childhood
   Anxiety states:
      Panic disorder—often begins in late adolescence
      Generalized anxiety disorder
      Obsessive compulsive disorder—usually beings in adolescence or early adulthood, but may begin in childhood
      Post-traumatic stress disorder—can occur at any age
Somatoform disorders (e.g., somatization disorder, conversion disorder, psychogenic pain disorder, hypocondriasis)
Psychosexual disorders
   Gender identity disorders:
      Transsexualism
      Gender identity disorder of childhood
      Paraphilias (e.g., exhibitionism, sexual masochism)
      Other psychosexual disorders (e.g., ego-dystonic homosexuality)
Factitious disorders
Disorders of impulse control not elsewhere classified (e.g., kleptomania, pyromania)
Adjustment disorder—may begin at any age
Personality disorders (Axis II of DSM-III)
   Although the symptoms of personality disorders may manifest themselves in adolescence or earlier, the diagnosis of a personality disorder (e.g., paranoid personality disorder, schizoid personality disorder, histrionic personality disorder, antisocial personality disorder) is generally reserved for adults. Some personality disorders in adults have a relationship to corresponding diagnostic categories for children or adolescents:

Disorders of childhood	Personality disorders
Schizoid disorder of childhood	Schizoid personality disorder
Avoidant disorder of childhood	Avoidant personality disorder
Conduct disorder (undersocialized, aggressive)	Antisocial personality disorder
Oppositional disorder	Passive-aggressive personality disorder
Identity disorder	Borderline personality disorder

[a]Although this list does include the more common children's mental disorders, it is not exhaustive. Furthermore, only selected disorders are discussed in the text of this background paper.
[b]Disorders in these classes are primarily adult diagnoses but may occur among children.

SOURCE: Adapted from American Psychiatric Association, *Diagnostic and Statistical Manual of Mental Disorders*, 3d ed. (Washington, DC: 1980).

infancy, childhood, or adolescence into five general categories based on the aspect of functioning that is most disturbed: intellectual, developmental, behavioral, emotional, and physical (psychophysiological). Examples of disorders in several of these categories are severe mental retardation, developmental reading disorder, undersocialized aggressive conduct disorder, reactive attachment disorder of infancy, chronic motor tic disorder, anorexia nervosa, encopresis, and enuresis.

In addition to the class of disorders that usually first become evident in children, several broad classes of mental disorders discussed in DSM-III may affect children. These classes and examples of disorders that may affect children are shown in table 6. Such disorders include substance use disorders, affective disorders such as major depression, various anxiety disorders, and adjustment disorder. Following DSM-III's heuristic for disorders that usually manifest themselves early in a person's life, substance use disorder is discussed in this background paper under behavior disorders, and depression and anxiety disorder under emotional disorders. Because it stems directly from an environmental stressor and can take various forms, adjustment disorder is discussed separately.

Any given child may have more than one DSM-III disorder, and disorders may involve problems across general categories. Furthermore, disturbances in one area are likely to have secondary effects on other areas of functioning. Thus, for example, a child with a specific developmental disorder will often have problems with behavior and emotions as a result.

Patterns of disturbance vary widely across diagnostic categories. Disturbances present different clinical patterns, pose different consequences for children and their families, impinge on different settings in varying ways, and require different treatments. Furthermore, mental disorders may vary in severity. In some cases, for example, childhood phobias are mild and transient; children often overcome such phobias in the course of development. In other cases, however, childhood phobias involve severe impairment and interfere in significant ways with a child's development (553). Beyond a certain level, the severity of a disorder must usually be assessed separately from the DSM-III diagnosis.

Several children's mental disorders within broad general categories are discussed below. The discussion is not exhaustive. The purpose is to give the reader a basic understanding of the range of childhood disorders, along with some information on their prevalence and their consequences for children. Most of the childhood disorders are reviewed, but a few are omitted in the interest of space because they are rare, their consequences are relatively less severe than those of other disorders, or because the disorders that are discussed sufficiently illustrate the broad category.

INTELLECTUAL DISORDERS

The only DSM-III mental disorder that primarily involves intellectual impairment is mental retardation, although secondary intellectual deficits are often involved in other disorders. Inclusion of mental retardation as a DSM-III mental disorder on Axis I has provoked concern.

One critical article (563) notes that mental retardation is primarily defined by a lowered *level* of intellectual functioning and thus differs from other disorders, which are characterized by abnormal *types* of functioning. Advocates for mentally retarded children seek to avoid any prejudice against this population stemming from the association of mental retardation with mental disorders (422). When mental retardation is discussed in this background paper, it is because of its inclusion in DSM-III or because many mentally retarded children have mental health treatment needs.

Mental retardation is defined as significantly subnormal intellectual ability that leads to deficits in functioning. In DSM-III, the criterion denoting intellectual ability in the mentally retarded range is a score on a standardized intelligence (IQ) test of 70 or below (although some flexibility on the IQ is allowed). IQ tests are standardized tests with a mean of 100 and a standard deviation of 15. A score of 70 is two standard deviations below the mean and places mentally retarded children in the bottom 2 percent of children intellectually.

There are an estimated 6 million mentally retarded persons in the United States; the range of intellectual impairment in these individuals is wide. The American Association on Mental Deficiency has identified four broad levels of mental retardation based on IQ: mild, moderate, severe, and profound (257). These levels are intended to correspond to the individual's capability for adaptive functioning and the degree to which training will result in independent functioning. In general, the more retarded an individual is, the less independence he or she can be expected to gain from training and the more supervision he or she will need for self-care, work, and social relationships. At the extreme, profoundly retarded individuals require a highly structured setting with continuous care. With adequate training, however, many mentally retarded individuals can function independently.

Most mentally retarded children—about 80 percent—are mildly retarded. Approximately 12 percent of retarded children are moderately retarded, 7 percent severely retarded, and 1 percent profoundly retarded (19).

Organic causation is not believed to be a factor in most mental retardation. Only about 25 percent of the incidence of mental retardation is attributable to organic causes (36); moderate, severe, and profound retardation are nearly always associated with organic brain damage. For 75 percent of mental retardation, almost all mildly retarded, however, there is no evidence of organic causation. How this type of mental retardation is caused is not well understood, but it is thought to stem from environmental causes, genetic causes, or a combination of the two.

Neurologically based impairments in coordination, vision, or hearing are often associated with mental retardation (19). Mentally retarded children are also three to four times more suscepti-

ble to other mental disorders than children in the general population (19), especially to other disorders that may have a neurological basis like stereotyped movement disorder and attention deficit disorder with hyperactivity (ADD-H) (19). They are at increased risk for problems with speech, language, and academic and social adjustment. Mental retardation can lead to stress, depression, and other emotional disturbances through several means. The parents of some mentally retarded children may reject or overprotect them (538), or mentally retarded children may gain awareness of their deficiencies, leading to low self-esteem and depression (538).

Further, mental retardation limits the number and quality of supportive relationships that children can form and limits their flexibility in solving problems; as a consequence, there is an increased likelihood that retarded children will be frustrated and adopt poor strategies for managing their lives. Institutionalized retarded children frequently manifest atypically heightened levels of dependency that are not attributable to cognitive level alone (730). The social environment of retarded children is apparently critical; whether they are institutionalized, placed in a community setting, or raised at home can affect their mental health. Similarly, their mental health can be enhanced by receiving education and training adapted to their abilities.

Care and training of the mentally retarded is generally handled by a special service system separate from the system that treats the emotionally or behaviorally disturbed. Moreover, it is not generally conceptualized by practitioners as mental health treatment. For these reasons, interventions specific to mental retardation are excluded from Parts III and IV of this background paper. The discussion of disorders, environmental risk factors, and services applies to mentally retarded children only insofar as such children have concomitant mental health problems. Because concomitant mental health problems are common in mentally retarded children, however, mental health treatment is an important part of the service needs of this population.

DEVELOPMENTAL DISORDERS

Developmental disorders are characterized by deviations from the normal path of child development. Such disorders can be either pervasive, affecting multiple areas of development, or specific, affecting only one aspect of development. Like mental retardation, developmental disorders pose multiple problems for a child. Pervasive developmental disorders (PDDs) severely limit children's ability to function independently, while specific developmental disorders (SDDs) can greatly impede children's education and development of social relations.

Pervasive Developmental Disorders (PDDs)

Children with a PDD experience severe deviations from normal development in a number of spheres. Primarily, these deviations are manifested in cognitive and intellectual functioning, language development, and social relationships. PDDs identified in DSM-III are infantile autism and childhood-onset PDD. DSM-III terms such as infantile autism or childhood-onset PDD have generally superseded older labels such as childhood schizophrenia or childhood psychosis.

Children with a PDD manifest a gross lack of interest in others and have problems relating, even to family members. They may appear oblivious to family members or caretakers walking in the room, as if they were inanimate. They often use language in bizarre ways—i.e., echoing what they are told, using phrases with their own private meaning or using the pronoun "you" to refer to themselves. Also, they often insist on the preservation of sameness in their environments and display odd finger movements or postures. PDD children vary in terms of specific symptoms (712), but they all share marked impairment. PDDs are relatively rare, but they affect somewhere between 50,000 and 100,000 children in the United States, approximately 1 per every 1,000 children (712).

The intellectual functioning of children with PDDs varies. Many of the children with a PDD are mentally retarded, and the majority are below average in intelligence. In extremely rare cases, children with a PDD have brilliant isolated skills, such as the ability to memorize train schedules or play musical instruments, although they may not be toilet trained or able to use language to communicate. The vast majority of children with a PDD require special educational programs, and many parents need professional consultation or training to deal with these difficult children (712).

In most cases, parents are able to care for PDD children at home, although home care can become increasingly difficult as the children become older (712). PDD is usually chronic, and the majority of affected individuals are permanently unable to function independently. Autistic adults are found in the same placements as adults who are mentally retarded or schizophrenic: hospitals, long-term residential treatment centers, boarding houses, and often their families' homes.

At one time, it was thought that the parents of PDD children rejected them or withdrew from them in such a way as to lead to disturbance in their development (58). Such ideas have generally been discredited. Studies indicate that there are no personality or other differences between parents of PDD children and other parents (97, 424). It is now suspected that PDD is related to impairment in neurochemistry or neuroanatomy.

Specific Developmental Disorders (SDDs)

Children with SDDs have difficulty with specific skills underlying learning, but their overall development is within normal ranges. DSM-III identifies several types of SDDs according to the particular skill which is impaired—e.g., developmental language disorders, developmental reading disorder (i.e., dyslexia), and developmental arithmetic disorder (19). In children with an SDD, the development of one of these specific skills is well below the average for the particular child's grade level. All SDDs combined are estimated to affect 3 to 5 percent of the school age population (41), although as much as 10 percent of the adult population is thought to have significant difficulties with reading, possibly related to an underlying disorder.

There are two forms of developmental language disorders: receptive type and expressive type. In the receptive type, children have trouble understanding spoken language; in the expressive type, children understand what they hear and know what they want to say, but have difficulty recalling and arranging the words necessary to speak. Developmental articulation disorder refers to pronunciation difficulties with English sounds such as "s" and "th," leading children to appear as if they are using "baby talk" (19). Developmental reading disorder and developmental arithmetic disorder are diagnosed when reading or arithmetic skills are impaired relative to expectations for a child's age, and neither deficits in intelligence nor schooling are deemed responsible.

SDD children are prone to school failure. Difficulties in learning are often compounded by secondary mental health problems, including school behavior problems, aggression or delinquency outside of school, anxiety and depression, and poor relationships with peers (41,576). The perceptual skills that are essential for learning to read, spell, write, and do arithmetic may also be important in social interactions and in establishing and maintaining social relationships (82,426).

In some cases, SDD children may have to endure the frustration and anger of parents and teachers who do not recognize their learning disability or understand how to help them. In such situations, parents or teachers may ascribe the child's failure to laziness or stubbornness. In certain cases, behavioral problems may partially cause the learning difficulty (576), but in other cases, emotional or behavioral problems stem from the breakdown in a child's education that is the consequence of having a learning disorder. Such secondary effects create additional obstacles to learning and reinforce a child's classroom failure (132). Many SDD children drop out of school in their teens (79).

BEHAVIOR DISORDERS

Behavior disorders are a set of problems in which a child's distress or disability is a function of his or her overt behavior. Since the central characteristics of these disorders are behaviors that disturb or harm others, the child's social environment plays a large part in whether that child will be identified as having behavior disorders and influences the course of these disorders. Some researchers and clinicians maintain that the nature of behavior disorders and the life history of affected children are especially dependent on the children's experience with social systems, such as the family, neighborhood, and school.

Attention Deficit Disorder (ADD)

Children with ADD are unable to maintain focused activity for more than a brief period and continually initiate new activities. Most children with ADD also suffer from hyperactivity, continual movement that is especially disruptive in structured group situations like a classroom. These children are diagnosed as having ADD with hyperactivity (ADD-H). In addition, there is a 50- to 80-percent overlap between ADD-H and some SDDs (462).

Schoolchildren with ADD may have great difficulty concentrating or inhibiting impulses to leave their seat and move around during class time. They may continually call out in class or push ahead of others in lines because they cannot tolerate waiting. Since the ability to maintain attention is essential to learning, children with ADD often have serious academic problems. Further problems may arise from the stress the child and school experience in dealing with the primary problem. Like SDD children, ADD children suffer from the frustration and poor self-image caused by not learning, the stigma of lagging behind their class, and the anger and frustration of parents and teachers. ADD children are prone to anxiety, depression, and social withdrawal (426), and typically have problems developing and maintaining friendships. The severity of ADD varies greatly across children (556). Some children are able to compensate for their difficulty with little interference in their lives, while others are so severely affected that they cannot tolerate normal school programs.

ADD children often exhibit aggressiveness or stubbornness and are prone to temper tantrums (439). Aggressiveness and impulsivity may be primary components of ADD, or they may be secondary consequences of the frustration and humiliation felt by a learning-disordered or hyperactive child. In addition, aggressiveness may arise from the struggle with teachers trying to deal with ADD children in the classroom.

An important factor in ADD is the ability of children's families and schools to tolerate and manage their behavior (470). Although it is unlikely that social factors cause hyperactivity, negative responses from the social environment toward these children are often an additional burden.

The outcome of ADD in adolescence and adulthood varies greatly. Some children seem to "outgrow" ADD, while others continue to suffer from ADD into adolescence and adulthood. In some cases, hyperactivity ends or attenuates in adolescence, but problems with distractibility or impulsivity often remain. As they grow to be adolescents and adults, hyperactive children have an increased risk of academic and behavioral problems, substance abuse, school failure, and contact with the legal system (62,306,435,441,692).

The causes of ADD are not well understood. It was once believed that ADD stemmed from prenatal or perinatal brain injury. But there is no evidence for the existence of brain damage among most affected children, and the difference between hyperactive and normal children in the birth process and infancy does not explain the existence of these disorders (556). Neurological differences between hyperactive children and normal children are plausible, but they may not reflect pathology so much as the general variation in cognitive abilities and temperament in children. Other research has implicated food additives, allergies, and environmental toxins as causal agents for hyperactivity (176,461), although such evidence is, at present, only suggestive.

Conduct Disorder

Children with conduct disorder exhibit a pattern of behavior that violates social norms, often harming others. Such children have a history of either infringement of the rights of others, or violations of the law, or both. Their pattern of misconduct includes behaviors such as fighting, vandalism, stealing, lying, rule-breaking, and running away from home. An ongoing history of misbehavior differentiates conduct disorders from the normal mischief of adolescence.

Conduct disorders are often first defined as problems by the legal system. Despite some overlap, however, conduct disorder is not the same as "juvenile delinquency." Conduct disorder is a psychiatric term describing a longstanding pattern of misbehavior, whereas delinquency is a legal term applied to minors convicted of an offense. Many children incarcerated in juvenile justice facilities would not be diagnosed as having conduct disorder, primarily because their behavior does not comprise a pattern. The extent to which juvenile crime is associated with actual conduct-disordered adolescents is unknown.

Children with conduct disorders differ in the degree to which they are socialized and capable of forming attachments to others, but there is controversy about whether differences in socialization constitute distinct types of conduct disorders (19). Some believe that adolescents who have good family and peer relationships, who have a reasonable sense of self, and whose delinquency primarily reflects neighborhood and peer group influence probably do not truly have a mental disorder (9). The antisocial behavior of such adolescents may be largely directed at those outside their gang or family.

Some children with conduct disorders are unable to form friendships or extend themselves to others in any way. These undersocialized behavior-disordered children relate to others in exploitive and egocentric ways. They are also likely to have experienced problems with conduct from an early age, when they would normally have developed the capacity to relate to others. Conduct disorders that begin prior to age 13 are particularly pernicious. Early onset often leads to serious consequences for both children with conduct disorders and people around them.

Although disorders of conduct are defined by a pattern of inappropriate behaviors, such disorders are often accompanied by considerable personal suffering, and children with conduct disorders usually have low self-esteem, despite outward bravado (19). These children often experience mental health problems such as depression, anxiety, or substance abuse, and/or have academic problems (19,565). Even when they are able to form significant relationships, the relationships may be fraught with conflict (432). It should also be noted that the occurrence of hyperactivity and conduct disorder overlaps considerably (624).

Estimates of the prevalence of conduct disorder vary greatly because of the use of different definitions of the disorder and different sources of data. In addition, the prevalence of conduct disorder varies depending on sociological variables such as low income and poor housing (703). General population surveys estimate the prevalence at 5 to 15 percent, but such surveys often use less stringent criteria than DSM-III (432). A further problem is that such surveys fail to distinguish between socialized and undersocialized children (432).

The course of conduct disorder depends greatly on social as well as individual factors (19). Gang-related delinquency, for example, depends on such factors as youth employment rates. Most children with conduct disorders, particularly those able to form relationships, are able to stop their misbehavior as they mature (546). Others may continue illegal behavior for financial gain, but function adequately otherwise. Many children with conduct disorders, however, continue their inappropriate behavior into adulthood and maintain a life centered around criminal behavior. They continue to have problems with social relationships, and many suffer in adulthood from alcoholism, drug dependence, or depression (544). These tend to be the children whose delinquency starts early and who have committed a greater number and variety of antisocial acts (544).

Many theories for explaining the development of conduct disorder implicate child-rearing practices. The parents of undersocialized, aggressive children are believed not to have formed a loving parental attachment to the infant. Many parents of children with conduct disorders are alcoholic or have a history of antisocial behavior (544,545). Often, children who develop conduct disorders are unwanted or unplanned. As the child matures, parents alternate between being uninterested in the child and being overly protective (432). Other theories suggest biological and genetic components to undersocialized conduct disorder (544).

Substance Abuse and Dependence

Drug and alcohol abuse are sometimes viewed as diseases separate from mental health problems. In terms of etiology and implications, however, substance abuse may be similar to other mental health difficulties. The implications of substance abuse for children and adolescents are particularly severe. Substance abuse broadly disrupts a young person's functioning, can cause distress and long-term disability, and can lead to or exacerbate conflict in family and peer relationships. Chronic drug and alcohol use can also harm academic and job performance. Legal problems arise both from actions carried out under the influence of drugs or alcohol and from buying, possessing, and selling drugs or alcohol. Several substances, such as alcohol, barbiturates and sedatives, opiates, and amphetamines, can, with frequent use, lead to chemical dependence.

Substance abuse is correlated with problems such as psychological distress (483), life stress (156), low school achievement (321), running away from home (160), parental drug use (547), and perceived lack of involvement by parents (483). Substance-abusing children are often troubled by anxiety and depressed moods (19). Several studies suggest that many adolescents who use alcohol and drugs heavily were psychologically disturbed as younger children (331,486,615; for conflicting evidence, 338). School learning problems and aggressive or antisocial behavior as a child are good predictors of later drug use, especially if they are associated with difficulties in relationships (338). Available evidence suggests that interventions aimed at treating substance abuse and dependence must also deal with the multitude of other mental health problems with which abusers are also afflicted (63).

Identifying substance abuse as a type of mental disorder is useful because it draws attention to the mental health implications of abusing chemical substances. Substance abuse in adolescents, however, is frequently associated with other mental disorders discussed in this chapter, including conduct disorder, ADD, and SDD. Substance use and abuse by children also illustrates the complexity of identifying discrete mental health problems and separating disorders from normal development. Considerable evidence suggests that substance use, and occasional abuse, is currently "a 'normal' developmental reality" among adolescents (369).

EMOTIONAL DISORDERS

Several children's mental disorders have their most noticeable effect on a child's emotional state. The severity of children's emotional problems varies widely. To represent a diagnosable mental disorder, however, an emotional problem must be accompanied by considerable impairment of a child's ability to function.

Anxiety Disorders

In children with anxiety disorders, excessive fearfulness and symptoms associated with fear interfere with a child's functioning. Anxiety-disordered children may experience muscular tension, have somatic complaints without physical basis, and experience repeated nightmares. Children with anxiety disorders may be preoccupied with unrealistic dangers and may avoid fear-producing situations to the point of stubbornness or tantrums.

Anxiety disorders that are especially associated with childhood or adolescence include separation anxiety disorder, avoidant disorder of childhood, overanxious disorder, and certain phobic disorders (19). Children with separation anxiety are afraid to be away from their parents, from home, or from familiar surroundings. They avoid a variety of normal activities and, in some cases, refuse to go to school. They may cling to parents and develop physical complaints when separation is about to occur; if separated, they become fearful, sometimes to the point of panic. Separation anxiety may lead children to have morbid fears about their parents' death, or difficulty sleeping if family members do not stay with them. This disorder often waxes and wanes during childhood years, usually increasing in response to stress.

Avoidant disorder of childhood or adolescence is similar in many ways to separation anxiety disorder, except that the focus of the problem is contact with strangers rather than separation from loved ones. These disorders rarely last beyond adolescence.

Phobias are irrational anxiety reactions to specific situations or objects leading children to avoid these situations or objects. Common childhood phobias include dog, school, and water phobias (553). Mild phobias are normal and occur among almost half of all children; they are usually outgrown. Phobias in an estimated 0.5 to 1 percent of children, however, can be intense and interfere with the child's development. Children avoid the feared object to the point of not participating in an important activity or avoiding learning important new behaviors. School phobia is perhaps the most common childhood phobia (553) and can lead to serious educational problems (343).

Childhood Depression

"Depression" can refer to a mood, to a set of related symptoms that occur together, or to a complete psychiatric disorder with characteristic symptoms, course, and prognosis (357). The psychiatric disorder includes both depressed mood and symptoms of impaired functioning such as insomnia, loss of appetite, slowed activity and speech, fatigue, self-reproach, diminished concentration, and suicidal or morbid thoughts (19).

Depression influences concentration, energy level, and confidence; can affect physical health; and is usually associated with a perhaps unrealistically pessimistic view of the world (367). Like other emotional disorders, it has the potential to seriously impair a child's abilities to function in school, with peers, and with family. Depressed children commonly withdraw from social relationships. The low self-regard, hopelessness, and helplessness of depressed adolescents may lead to suicide (93). The amount of mental suffering depressed children undergo can be considerable, although the degree of impairment and length of the depression vary considerably (19).

Many depressed children exhibit behavioral problems that are more longstanding and more alarming to adults than their depression (95). A conduct or learning problem may be labeled as the chief disturbance that needs treatment, while their depression is overlooked. Some theorists and researchers have called this "masked" depression, because these behavioral difficulties, in their ability to stir up and distract the child and others, protect the child from experiencing painful, depressed feelings (133). Recent research, however, suggests that with careful questioning, many such children with behavioral problems will reveal pervasive problems with mood as well as behavior (102).

Depressive symptoms specific to children may occur, including anxiety over separation from parents, clinging, and refusal to go to school. Depressed adolescents may react with sulky, angry, or aggressive behavior; problems in school; or substance abuse (19). Estimates of the prevalence of childhood depression are variable as a result of differing criteria used by researchers, differences in the age of children studied, and other differences among the populations examined (333). Estimates range from 0.14 percent (564) to 1.9 percent (332). Among children brought to psychiatric or education-related treatment centers, estimates range as high as 59 percent (505). Available research does not permit an overall conclusion about the incidence and prevalence of childhood depression or about the relationship of childhood depression to other disorders.

The large number and range of theories suggesting the cause of depression are notable. What seems most likely is that psychological, biological, and social causal factors arise together to initiate and perpetuate depression (13). Most models

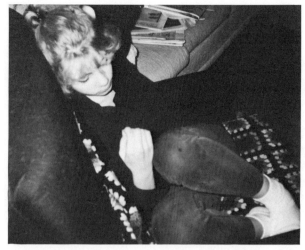

Photo credit: OTA

It is sometimes difficult to distinguish between common adolescent emotional turmoil and more serious forms of childhood depression and anxiety.

used in explaining how childhood depression develops are borrowed from analyses of adult depression. Studies assessing the applicability of adult models to childhood depression have been conducted only recently. For example, much evidence substantiates the relationship between depression in adults and low concentrations of certain neurotransmitters (biochemicals that provide for transmission of impulses across nerve cells). Several studies have found lower levels of the by-products of these neurotransmitters in the urine of children with chronic depressive disorder (428).

Even when children are not clinically depressed, persistent poor mood or symptoms such as insomnia or poor appetite often accompany other childhood disorders or stressful situations or events. Clinicians treating children must often attend to the depressed mood which accompanies demoralization felt in the face of a number of the other disorders, or environmental or medical stressors.

Reactive Attachment Disorder of Infancy

Reactive attachment disorder of infancy, in some severe cases called "failure to thrive," denotes a syndrome in which infants who are receiving inadequate care are poorly developed both emotionally and physically. If the disorder is not treated, it often results in severe physical complications: malnutrition, starvation, or even death. Case studies also show that failure to thrive can lead to feeding disorders such as obsession with food and food refusal.

Reactive attachment disorder exemplifies the complexity of the origins of childhood mental health problems. DSM-III states: "The diagnosis of Reactive Attachment Disorder of Infancy can be made only in the presence of clear evidence of lack of adequate care" (19). Often, however, the disorder does not arise simply from "bad" parenting, but instead arises from a combination of both complications in an infant's development and emotional difficulties and stress affecting parents (153). Some parents interpret problems in an infant's feeding or development as rejection. If a parent, as a result, is unable to properly interpret an infant's cues to be fed, the infant will not be fed adequately, and may develop a severe reactive attachment disorder. Parents who have emotional difficulties or are burdened with stress are especially predisposed to such a response. A pattern of similar breakdowns in communication between infants and parents can also lead to difficulties developing emotional attachments between parents and children, and later with the child's developing appropriate autonomy. Yet reactive attachment disorder of infancy can be "completely reversed" by adequate care (19).

PSYCHOPHYSIOLOGICAL DISORDERS

Children's mental disorders that involve a disturbance in some aspect of bodily functioning usually involve a combination of mental and physical factors; hence, these disorders have been called psychophysiological disorders. Psychophysiological disorders include stereotyped movement disorders, enuresis and encopresis, and eating disorders. As described below, the physical manifestations of psychophysiological disorders are diverse. These disorders may place children at great risk, since they pose threats to both physical and mental health.

Stereotyped Movement Disorders

Stereotyped movement disorders are thought to have a primary physical or neurological basis. Nevertheless, such disorders are influenced by the psychological state of the child and are sometimes amenable to behavioral or psychological intervention.

Children with stereotyped movement disorders suffer from tics—sudden, repetitive movements of a particular body part. In a rare form of stereotyped movement disorder, Tourette's syndrome, vocal tics (short grunts, yelps, or other vocal sounds) accompany the body movements (19). Tics are generally involuntary, although they can be suppressed temporarily through concentration (19,598). In general, they are thought to have an organic basis, yet stress or anticipation can increase their frequency (314,598). Tics may be a transient or chronic problem (19). Although 12 to 24 percent of schoolchildren in surveys have reported having had tics at some time, overall prevalence is unknown because there is no information on how many children have this difficulty at any one time. Children with these disorders suffer considerable embarrassment and are often unable to bring their tics under continual voluntary control. These disorders sometimes disappear in adulthood, but can be lifelong.

Eating Disorders

Disorders involving eating behavior include a varied group of dysfunctions. The most common eating disorders are anorexia nervosa and bulimia, which occur primarily in adolescents. Anorexia is characterized by a refusal to eat, leading to a loss of body weight (literally, "nervous weight loss"). The DSM-III diagnosis of anorexia nervosa applies to those who have lost at least 25 percent of body weight. Individuals with this disorder, typically adolescent girls and young women, starve themselves because of an exaggerated fear that they will be overweight and therefore unattractive.

In extreme cases, children with anorexia nervosa may refuse to eat altogether, even if they are already very thin. Because of the possibility of malnutrition, serious medical illness, or death, anorexia can have serious consequences. Psychological complications such as depression and withdrawal can also result from the starvation involved with anorexia nervosa. These complications often overshadow the original psychiatric problems that led to the eating disorder (620).

Bulimia is, in some respects, the converse of anorexia nervosa. Bulimics, usually adolescents, consume large quantities of food in one sitting ("binge eating"). They often stop only when pain or nausea is too great to continue. Often, bulimics self-induce vomiting or use laxatives, enemas, or diuretics to purge themselves of what they have eaten. Because of the physical insult of this pattern of behavior, bulimia can be associated with physiological disturbance. Although the prevalence of bulimia in adolescents is unknown (19), recent surveys (271,626) indicate an incidence rate of 13 to 67 percent for self-reported binge eating in college populations. Such data suggest that the problem of bulimia is substantial, although it may most frequently appear only as a transient problem. Various adjustment problems often accompany a bulimic disorder, including depression and difficulty with social relationships (322,335,708).

Perhaps the most serious eating disorder is the coincidence of the two above disorders, which has been called "bulimarexia" (64). Affecting primarily adolescents, bulimarexia combines obsessive self-denial of food with intermittent binge eating. Casper and her colleagues (105) found that almost half of a sample of patients with anorexia also suffered from bulimia, and that these patients were significantly more obsessional about food, more guilty, more depressed, and more likely to be involved in compulsive stealing.

Enuresis and Encopresis

Enuresis is the diagnostic term for bedwetting and other inappropriate urination, while encopresis is the term for lack of control over defecation. Each of these disorders has relationships to other disorders as well as complicated connections to physiology, environmental factors, and family genetic history. In many cases, physical problems either cause these disorders or predispose children to them (19,596), and there is some evidence that enuresis tends to run in families (19,33). But enuresis and encopresis tend to occur more frequently in disadvantaged families (440), under stressful conditions (19,523), and together with other disorders (565). Enuresis affects 5 to 15 percent of 7-year-olds (565) and encopresis 1 percent of 5-year-olds (19).

ADJUSTMENT DISORDER

For most DSM-III disorders, a cause is not specified, because in most cases, causes of disorders are as yet unknown (19). Adjustment disorder, however, refers to a pattern of emotional or behavioral difficulties that occurs in response to a stressful event. Stressful events can overwhelm the capacity of children to cope, leading them to develop disabling emotional reactions to the stress or to develop unfortunate ways of trying to cope that create more problems. Stressful events leading to adjustment disorder could include any of a variety of crises such as divorce or acute illness of a parent. Adjustment disorder often remits without treatment, either because the stressful life event has ended or because the child and family have developed new resources equal

to the stress. In vulnerable children and families, however, an adjustment disorder can usher in more serious difficulties.

The main features of adjustment disorder are depressed or anxious moods, antisocial behavior (especially in adolescents), difficulties that infants have in their interaction with their primary caregivers, or inability to work or maintain relationships (19). Thus, adjustment disorder resembles psychiatric disorders such as anxiety disorder or conduct disorder. Adjustment disorder is differentiated from disorders with parallel symptoms on the basis of how long the problem has lasted and whether or not it followed from a stressful event. The diagnosis of adjustment disorder is sometimes made by child clinicians because they would often rather use the more benign label of adjustment disorder than diagnoses such as conduct disorder or major depression which imply more pervasive impairment.

CONCLUSION

The five general categories of children's mental disorders discussed in this chapter—intellectual, developmental, behavioral, emotional, and psychophysiological—represent patterns of dysfunctional adaptation in children. Although normal, as well as mentally disordered, children may exhibit symptoms of these disorders, in each case, it is the pattern of pervasive difficulty that leads to the diagnosis. No mental disorder, however well-described by current psychiatric nomenclature, manifests itself in parallel ways across children. Environmental risk factors, to be discussed in chapter 4, can influence both the manifestation and course of children's mental disorders. In addition, when maladjustment of a child occurs, it does not necessarily take the form of mental disability as defined by psychiatric nomenclature.

The diversity and complexity of children's mental health problems suggests a need for treatment approaches differentiated according to each specific child's needs. In addition, the relationship of many of these problems to normal functioning suggests a need for integrating mental health services with family and school settings in which children function. Subsequent chapters of this background paper consider these topics more explicitly.

Environmental Risk Factors and Children's Mental Health Problems

Chapter 4
Environmental Risk Factors and Children's Mental Health Problems

INTRODUCTION

As decribed in chapter 3, diagnostic manuals, such as the American Psychiatric Association's *Diagnostic and Statistical Manual* (DSM-III), define mental disorders and set out criteria that must be met for a mental health problem to be considered a disorder. In DSM-III (19), a mental health problem is considered a disorder only if the problem is:

> . . . a clinically significant behavioral or psychological syndrome or pattern . . . that is typically associated with a painful symptom (distress) or impairment in one or more areas of functioning.

Although defining and establishing criteria for mental disorders is useful, it can mean that children with subclinical mental health problems, or those in danger of developing a disorder, may not be considered to be in need of mental health services. In reality, children, particularly those exposed to environmental stressors, may exhibit discrete mental health problems. For example, a child whose parents divorce may experience anger and depression. Children with a major physical illness may experience loneliness when they cannot see their family and friends. Children born into or thrust into poverty may experience constant anxiety as a result of financial insecurity. Further, some children are exposed to multiple stressors and so may be vulnerable to a number of mental health problems.

The multiaxial system of DSM-III incorporates environmental stressors on Axis IV (psychosocial stressors, including stress arising from physical illness) (19; also see ch. 3). Because DSM-III is primarily a manual for clinicians, however, it necessarily treats psychosocial stressors as additional, rather than primary, information to be used in developing a mental health treatment plan for a patient. Although there is disagreement about the value of primary prevention of mental health problems (15), it is widely agreed that it may be possible to address certain environmental stressors preventively.

This chapter describes a number of environmental stressors that children may be exposed to, along with the mental health problems that may be caused or exacerbated by such stressors. The chapter does not review every environmental factor that poses a risk to children's mental health, but it does attempt to cover the specific environmental, primarily psychosocial, factors that pose the greatest risk and to illustrate generally the effect that environment can have on the development of children's mental health problems. And, as acknowledged by DSM-III's multiaxial diagnostic system, these environmental factors can also affect the course of mental health problems, and plans to treat such problems. Discussed are poverty; premature birth; parental psychopathology such as alcoholism, maltreatment, teenage parenting (a problem for both parent and child); and parental divorce. The purposes are to focus attention on the range of children's mental health problems that may be amenable to intervention, whether the intervention is designed to alleviate pain or prevent development of more severe problems; and to raise the issue that it seems essential to develop policies and programs so that they work for the particular children who need to be helped. As discussed in chapter 2, several national commissions have stressed the importance of attending to environmental factors in developing mental health programs for children. These commissions have also made specific suggestions for developing such policies and programs. However, it is beyond the scope of this background paper to draw out fully all the implications of designing a mental health services system so that it is responsive to all the children in need.

INTERACTIONS AMONG ENVIRONMENTAL RISK FACTORS

Single environmental risk factors rarely occur in isolation. Much more common is the occurrence of several risk factors together—often in the context of a broad risk factor such as low socioeconomic status. Child maltreatment, for example, most often occurs in families that are disorganized, under high stress, and of low socioeconomic status (219,499,500). Parental divorce often results in downward economic mobility, relocation to more stressful circumstances, increased social isolation, and loss of important support systems (289).

For a comprehensive look at the mental health needs of children, it is important to consider how risk factors interact with one another. For example, ethnicity, social class, and related variables (e.g., years of parent education) have been found to have a powerful influence on a child's development. They, in turn, are related to parental attitudes towards childrearing (360, 572); to the quality of parent-child interaction (640); to children's cognitions, motivations, personality, and achievement behavior (144,149,150,241,287,320,392,732); and, of course, to the community in which a child lives and the school he or she attends.

It is also important to consider children's difficulties in the context of knowledge about normal development. It is useful to describe the negative effects of environmental risk factors in terms of a child's difficulties with completing important developmental tasks. Developmental tasks are the activities children engage in so as to advance to the next stage of their development (e.g., becoming toilet-trained is a developmental task for toddlers; developing intense friendships with peers is a developmental task for young adolescents). A child's failure to carry out salient developmental tasks can appropriately be viewed as an indicator of maladjustment.

POVERTY AND MEMBERSHIP IN A MINORITY ETHNIC GROUP

Being poor and being a member of a minority group are environmental stressors that may pose risks to children's mental health (116). Although it is important to recognize that most poor and minority individuals make health adjustments (116), the relationships between these environmental risk factors and poor social and psychological functioning is well recognized (15). In their 1981 review of the epidemiologic literature on the prevalence of mental disorders in children, for example, Gould, et al. (248), noted that children who were poor, black, or Spanish-speaking and living in an urban environment had mental health problems at rates greater than the 11.8 percent found in U.S. communities on average. Although the relationships are correlational rather than causal, increasing evidence about the effects of psychosocial stress on both physical and mental health supports the view that poverty and minority status pose risks for mental health (15). In addition, poverty and minority status are often accompanied by other risk factors, making children

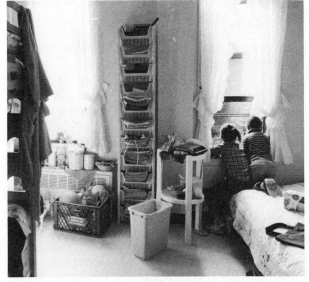

Photo credit: New York Times/Peter Freed

Children who must live in shelters may be at increased risk of developing mental health problems as a result of adverse environmental factors such as poverty, unstable home life, and inadequate care.

exposed to other risk factors even more vulnerable to developing mental health problems.

The relationship of socioeconomic class and ethnicity to mental health takes on particularly great importance with evidence that poverty among children—especially among black and Hispanic children—has increased in recent years. A report prepared by the Congressional Research Service and the Congressional Budget Office indicates that in 1983 there were 13.8 million poor children in the United States (646). The report

notes that child poverty rates have increased sharply among black and Hispanic children. Currently, almost half of black children in the United States live in poverty, while less than 15 percent of nonblack children are poor (117). Being poor may also mean that children will not have access to health insurance. An estimated 15.9 million children and young adults (1- to 19-year-olds) were uninsured in 1977, the last year for which national data are available (661a).

PARENTAL PSYCHOPATHOLOGY

In most children's development, the family plays a crucial role. It is perhaps not surprising, therefore, that the presence in the family of a parent with psychopathology increases a child's risk of experiencing emotional and behavioral difficulties. Some of the difficulties that the children of mentally ill parents may develop meet the criteria for standard DSM-III psychiatric diagnoses; other difficulties, however, are general impairments in children's social, emotional, or cognitive functioning that do not meet the standard criteria for diagnosable mental disorders. The relative contribution of genetic and environmental factors in causing the emotional and behavioral difficulties of children with mentally ill parents is not clear. Nonetheless, the occurrence of mental illness in a parent constitutes a significant risk factor to a child's psychological well-being.

Affectively Disordered Parent

The development of children who have a parent with an affective disorder, such as depression or manic-depressive illness, has been a focus of much research. Evidence about the incidence of affective disorders within families indicates that 10 to 40 percent of the immediate relatives of affectively disordered individuals also develop such disorders (225,315,501,613,713). There is growing awareness that children can manifest the symptoms of affective illness; although manic-depression is found infrequently in children and young adolescents, depression does exist during childhood (95).

Considering the effects of affectively disordered parents on their children is important, because affective disorders—particularly depression—are the major form of psychopathology to which children are exposed. The incidence of diagnosable depression in adult women has been estimated at 1 to 8 percent (70), and an even higher proportion (20 to 25 percent) are estimated to manifest marked, untreated depressive symptoms (69). Further, the presence of infants and young children in the home increases the risk for depression in adult women (45,695).

In children of affectively ill parents, DSM-III disorders as diverse as depression, separation anxiety, attention deficit disorder, personality disturbances, and conduct disorder have been identified (371,560,697). The overall prevalence of diagnosable mental disorders in these children has been found to be in the vicinity of 40 percent (428,467,477). Although the rates found in various studies are not directly comparable (because of the use of different diagnostic criteria), the similar direction of results confirms that the children of affectively ill parents have a higher incidence of depression and other problems than the children of normal parents.

Parental depression and mania seem to have a particularly marked effect on cognitive and emotional development during infancy and early childhood (115,218,571,696,725). Studies comparing the effects of maternal depression with those of schizophrenia (572), and the effects of maternal "psychological unavailability," often a result of depression, with those of physical abuse and neglect (162) for example, indicate that a mother's affective illness has a particularly pathogenic effect on a child's early development. In one study, children of psychologically unavailable mothers evidenced striking declines in functioning in every important area of development from birth to 2 years (162). As a group, these children appeared even more impaired than children exposed to physical abuse and neglect.

In middle childhood, children of affectively disordered parents often experience difficulty in important developmental tasks. Such children have been found to exhibit problems in meeting norms of school and classroom behavior (192,688); poor academic performance (550,551); and difficulty with peers, especially in terms of aggressive behavior (689).

As adolescents, the children of affectively disordered parents often experience difficulties that are more severe than those of other children. Garmezy and Devine (221) found, for example, that children of depressed mothers drop out of junior high school at more than twice the rate of controls (22 v. 10 percent).

Studies of children of parents with affective impairments have looked almost exclusively at mothers; therefore it is difficult to draw conclusions about children of fathers with affective impairments.

Schizophrenic Parent

A parent with schizophrenia, a debilitating and often chronic mental disorder, places a child at serious risk for developing mental health problems. Persons who are schizophrenic are plagued by hallucinations, delusions, or other thought disturbances. Children of schizophrenic parents have been shown to have a risk of developing schizophrenia 10 times greater than that of the offspring of nonschizophrenic parents (246). In general, these children also have more difficulties during childhood than do children of nonschizophrenic parents (682). This observation holds true even in the case of children who have not spent the majority of their childhoods living with the schizophrenic parent.

Prior to birth, the children of a schizophrenic mother may already have experienced more adverse circumstances than the children of nonschizophrenic mothers. The pregnancies and deliveries of schizophrenic mothers are more frequently accompanied by complications than those of nonschizophrenic mothers (430,431,571,720), and such complications are frequently related to children's developmental problems. Some researchers have found the increased pregnancy and birth complications of schizophrenic mothers to be associated with the low socioeconomic status that often accompanies schizophrenia (571), while others have found them to be independent (720).

In infancy and early childhood, children of a schizophrenic parent often exhibit a number of mental health difficulties. Such children often score lower than other children on measures of cognitive, linguistic, and psychomotor functioning, and they evidence deficiencies in adaptive behavior and emotional attachment (571). These problems can be exacerbated by the severity and chronicity of the illness and the low socioeconomic status typically associated with schizophrenia (571,572).

During the preschool and early elementary school years, children of a schizophrenic parent generally do not exhibit severe behavior problems. During middle childhood, however, evidence of serious social and academic difficulties emerge when these children are compared to the children of nonschizophrenic parents. Children of schizophrenics are rated by teachers and by peers as less competent than other children (550). These lower ratings of competence seem to stem from a perception of these children as more aggressive, impulsive, and disruptive (431,687). Furthermore, children of schizophrenics seem to have serious difficulties in terms of intellectual functioning. In comparison to the children of nonschizophrenic parents, they tend to have lower grades (551), lower IQ scores (431,460,717), and less scholastic motivation (316). In addition, these children have been found to exhibit more attentional dysfunction (460), more emotional instability (316,683), and a greater amount of psychological disturbance in general (718).

In most studies on the development of children of schizophrenics, subjects have not yet reached the age at which schizophrenia becomes manifest (i.e., the early twenties). Nonetheless, they already appear vulnerable. Although epidemiologic research suggests that only 10 percent of the children of schizophrenics themselves develop schizophrenia in adulthood, one study found that 75 percent of these high-risk children develop some form of psychiatric disturbance (295).

The relative contributions of genetic and environmental factors in schizophrenia are not known. It is also unclear whether the negative psychological impact of having a schizophrenic parent is due to the features of the disorder, to factors related to mental illness generally (e.g., severity and chronicity), or to the lower socioeconomic status that usually accompanies this major form of psychopathology.

Alcoholic Parent

Alcoholism is one of our Nation's most serious health problems (648,581), and the prevalence of alcoholism and alcohol abuse among adult men and women (up to 15 percent) suggests that parental alcoholism is one of the most common hazards to children's mental health. Abuse of illegal drugs by parents has also been implicated in the etiology of drug abuse by children (668a), but has not been subject to as much analysis as has parental alcohol abuse.

Approximately 6.6 million children under the age of 18 in the United States are estimated to have an alcoholic parent (559). That alcoholism may have serious negative effects on child-rearing and family relations is suggested by the well-documented harmful consequences of alcoholism to health, productivity, and other aspects of adult functioning (see 648). Alcoholism can disable parents from caring for their children effectively, and

it is associated with a n problems that place childre ness. Such problems include tion and divorce, violence, an as job loss and frequent moves

One of the earliest consequences parental alcoholism is the exposure of the fetus to alcohol (1). Evidence suggests that alcoholic mothers have increased risk of complications in pregnancy and of having children who develop health problems such as physical anomalies (e.g., heart defects) and disturbances to physical growth (165). Development of fetal alcohol syndrome, with a combination of birth defects, deficiency in growth, and deficits in development, is rare (165), but the development of fetal alcohol effects may be more common.

The disinhibiting effect of alcohol suggests that alcoholism may be associated with child abuse, although literature examining this relationship is equivocal (165,166). Some researchers find increased prevalence of alcoholism among child abusers, others find no relationship, while still others find that psychosocial disorders in general, including alcoholism, are associated with child abuse.

Only a few studies have examined the effect of parental alcoholism on children's development, despite frequent clinical suggestions about the damaging effects of family alcoholism on a child's personality and family relationships (685). Some studies have identified children of alcoholics as more susceptible than other children to a range of psychological, educational, and social problems including "emotional disturbance," hyperactivity, legal problems and drug abuse as adolescents, and a variety of behavioral problems and psychiatric disorders (165,166). However, it is difficult to rule out the possibility that related factors such as socioeconomic status or family disorganization are producing these effects.

MALTREATMENT

Recent estimates suggest that each year over 1 million children experience some type of maltreatment (662). "Maltreatment" includes physical in-

jury, sexual abuse, neglect and failure to provide, and emotional mistreatment. An estimated 100,000 to 200,000 children each year experience physi-

.ouse, 60,000 to 100,000 experience sexual ..use, and over 700,000 children are neglected (57). Although there are no estimates of the prevalence of emotional maltreatment, it is logical to assume that emotional maltreatment accompanies other forms of maltreatment and that there is another unknown number of children who experience emotional maltreatment alone. Maltreated children are often exposed to more than one type of maltreatment (162,231,284). Furthermore, maltreatment often consists of more than a single episode; studies suggest that approximately half of maltreated children have experienced previous abuse (159,282,377,610,737).

Maltreatment has long been thought to constitute a significant risk factor for children's development. Recent clinical and empirical investigations of maltreated children substantiate this assumption. The quality of available research varies (see 3); however, the research suggests that maltreated children are at high risk for physical, cognitive, behavioral, and emotional difficulties. Recent research and theorizing about maltreatment, although inadequate (see 729), documents the cognitive and social-emotional problems of maltreated children.

Physical Abuse and Neglect

Physical abuse and neglect are believed to cause intellectual and cognitive deficits, specifically lowered IQ scores that are frequently in the mentally retarded range. Clinical investigations of physically maltreated infants and children report that large numbers of these children are functioning at diminished cognitive and intellectual levels. Research suggests that 33 to 57 percent of physically abused and neglected infants and children have IQ scores below 85 (168,413,416,448).

Physically abused and neglected infants have been shown to have diminished performance on IQ tests and other developmental measures compared to a retrospective control group (23,146, 194,256,366). Comparison group studies of the cognitive and academic functioning of preschoolers and older children have frequently found that abused and neglected children perform at significantly lower levels than similar, nonmaltreated children (39,194,212,302,344,502). However, most of these studies are correlational, and it is possible that at least some children may be targets of abuse because of cognitive deficits.

In early and middle childhood, maltreated children exhibit several signs of social and emotional maladjustment. As preschoolers, maltreated children exhibit more adjustment problems and behavioral symptoms indicative of pathology (163, 502). They are also described as more aggressive, especially in response to frustration (283). As school-aged children, they frequently have impaired self-concepts and display heightened levels of aggression, both with peers and in the classroom (66,302,534,535). There is also limited evidence of self-destructive behaviors in these children, including suicide attempts, threats and gestures, and self-mutilative behavior (255). Finally, in their interaction with adult strangers, maltreated children are found to be more dependent and imitative than other children, and to exhibit less motivation to shape their own lives and make their own decisions (2). It has been hypothesized that these tendencies negatively affect maltreated children's ability to cope with the important developmental tasks of entry into school and effective functioning in the classroom.

That physical abuse and neglect causes at least some such deficits in development is supported by studies that compared maltreated children to control groups that are similar on important demographic and socioeconomic variables. The use of a matched, nonmaltreated control group is particularly important, since abuse and neglect often occur in the context of other risk factors such as high-stress environments and reduced socioeconomic status (222,228,499). Studies using control groups suggest that maltreatment causes cognitive deficits, in terms of both performance on IQ tests and academic functioning in school.

Studies using comparison groups also substantiate clinical observations that a significant degree of social and emotional maladaptation results from a history of physical maltreatment. As infants and toddlers, physically maltreated children are often insecurely attached to their caregivers (162,584), a factor that has been related to social and emotional difficulties throughout early childhood (385,421,623). In interactions with caregivers, physically maltreated infants and toddlers frequently exhibit withdrawal; inconsistency and unpredictability in affective communication; a lack of pleasure; indiscriminate attachment (214); and high levels of frustration, noncompliance, and aggression (162).

Although the relationship between cognitive performance and emotional difficulties in physically abused children is not clear, emotional and behavioral problems exhibited by maltreated children have been well documented. Clinical reports of physically maltreated infants and children describe a heterogeneous group of behavioral and emotional difficulties. These include severe anxiety, withdrawal, apathy in social interactions, and hypervigilance and "frozen watchfulness" in regard to the social environment (217,414,415,479, 634). In addition, these children are described as aggressive, oppositional, impulsive, provocative, and limit-testing (254,414,415). They exhibit a variety of other behavioral symptoms (e.g., hyperactivity, sleep disturbances, and socially inappropriate behavior), as well as significant sadness, low self-esteem, and self-depreciating behaviors (254,414,415).

Sexual Abuse

It has been estimated that 60,000 to 100,000 children are sexually abused in the United States every year (659), although some observers believe that available estimates probably represent only a small percentage of actual cases (18). This belief is supported by surveys of adults in which 15 to 34 percent report having been sexually victimized as children (191). In general, girls are sexually abused more frequently than boys, and the offender is often a family member, particularly a father or stepfather (122,191,453). Much less is known about the effects of sexual abuse on a child's mental health than is known about the effects of physical abuse and neglect. Nonetheless,

psychological and psychiatric literature strongly suggest that the experience of sexual victimization in childhood has serious deleterious psychological effects, both short and long term.

One study of the short-term effects of sexual abuse in children (12) found that all of the affected children and adolescents were symptomatic and in need of mental health attention. The degree of pathology ranged from mild to severe (e.g., anxiety and sleep disturbances, suicidal ideation, adjustment reactions, psychoses). In general, emotional disturbance was greater when the child was female, was unsupported by a close adult, had been molested by a father and/or by more than one relative, and had been genitally molested. Severity of disturbance was associated both with longstanding abuse that began in early childhood and with sexual abuse in adolescence, even if limited to only one incident.

One review of the literature indicates that sexually abused children and adolescents suffer from problems with sexual adjustment, interpersonal relationships, and educational functioning (452). The review suggests that when no disclosure or effective intervention occurs, difficulties can persist into adulthood. The most prominent effects of child sexual abuse found in adult populations are disturbed self-esteem and an inability to develop trust in intimate relationships (191).

Unfortunately, available research does not allow us to determine the degree to which these emotional and other psychological difficulties are due to sexual abuse or to other factors in the environment. Features of sexual abuse that seem most strongly related to negative psychological impact include the nature of the offense, the degree to which the offender is known, the use of force, and the age of the offender (190,227,373). Increased public recognition of problems engendered by sexual abuse is leading to better identification of the psychological effects and implications for treatment.

TEENAGE PARENTING

Adolescent parenthood has received increasing attention in recent years as the perception of the frequency and magnitude of this phenomenon has

grown. Of the over 3 million live births that occur annually in the United States, approximately 600,000 are to adolescent girls between 15 and 19

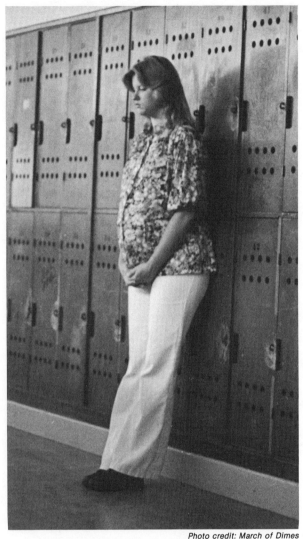

Approximately 600,000 of the 3 million births that occur annually are to adolescent girls between 15 and 19 years of age.

years of age (627). Additionally, an estimated 30,000 girls under age 14 become pregnant each year, of whom approximately 36 percent (10,800) give birth (558).

Teenage mothers are often from families of low socioeconomic status and low educational levels (111,669). Half of adolescent mothers do not complete high school (120). Approximately 17 percent of teenage mothers become pregnant again during the year following the birth of a first child; a second teenage pregnancy is more likely among adolescents from poor families (200). The vast majority of teenage mothers are unwed at the time of conception (465,726); in 1980 to 1981, only one-third of teenage mothers were married before the birth of their first child (466). The proportion of children born to unwed mothers has doubled since the early 1960s, and unwed mothers today are less likely to marry after the birth of a child than were unwed mothers in prior decades (466). The unwed mothers who do marry are more likely to divorce (213,393,578).

Teenage pregnancy and childbearing are associated with heightened medical risks to both mother and child. In girls younger than 15 years, in particular, there is a reduced likelihood of receiving adequate prenatal care, and an increased probability of morbidity and mortality in the offspring and toxemia in the mother (76,446,558). Offspring of teenage mothers have a greater probability of being premature and of low birthweight than those born to older mothers (427). In addition, there is an increased incidence of neurological abnormalities in the infants of teenage mothers (73,123,188). Teenage mother-infant dyads are characterized by less than optimal behaviors; these are often found to be associated with lower scores on tests of the infant's motor and mental development (183,409,573).

Cognitive deficits and diminished academic performance have been found in the preschool and school-aged children of teenage mothers. Children born to teenage mothers have been found to perform more poorly than other children on standardized IQ and achievement tests and on assessments of preparation for school (52,213,409). In one study, first-grade children who were born to adolescents were rated by their teachers as "less likely to adapt to school," a variable that correlates strongly with psychiatric symptoms in the teenage years (339).

In assessing the impact of low parental age on children's development, it is important to note the influence of other environmental factors. The most important of these are low socioeconomic status and marital instability. Both social disadvantage and marital instability have powerful effects on the development of children, independent of the effects attributable to maternal age.

Substantial evidence suggests that many of the negative effects of teenage parenting are only minimally related to the mother's age at birth, and are instead a function of the parent's reduced educational achievement and low socioeconomic status (35). Adolescent mothers have been found to have relatively limited knowledge and unrealistic expectations about child development (142). Some research indicates an association between adolescent parenting and child abuse (401,608, 617). In general, better outcomes on a range of indicators (e.g., cognitive skills) are found for adolescent mothers and their children who are receiving more support either from the children's father or from the mother's family compared with those in which the mother is the sole, full-time caretaker (213).

PREMATURE BIRTH AND LOW BIRTHWEIGHT

Premature birth (defined as gestational age of less than 37 weeks) and low birthweight (weight less than 2,500 grams) have potentially broad effects on mental health functioning. The incidence of prematurity is higher among infants born to mothers of low socioeconomic status than among other infants (478,541) and is approximately 10 percent for white infants and 20 percent for black infants (403).

The strong association of socioeconomic status and race with prematurity and low birthweight is probably due in part to the association of these variables with other important factors affecting neonatal status—e.g., the age of the mother, the mother's previous pregnancy history, and the availability of prenatal care for mother and infant (391). Given the associations between preterm birth and social and economic circumstances, it is often difficult to separate the effects of prematurity from effects related to the correlates of premature birth (e.g., social and economic circumstances and other illnesses in the child). Moreover, the developmental outcome of premature infants is being affected by medical advances that increase the survival rate of smaller and younger infants (210).

At present, prematurely born infants are likely to experience some difficulties in several domains of functioning, including social, environmental, linguistic, physical, and cognitive areas. One of the earliest difficulties to appear is disturbed interactions between mothers and preterm infants. These disturbances constitute a pattern of the infant showing less responsiveness, less positive affect, and more aversion behaviors than full-term infants and the mother showing more than the

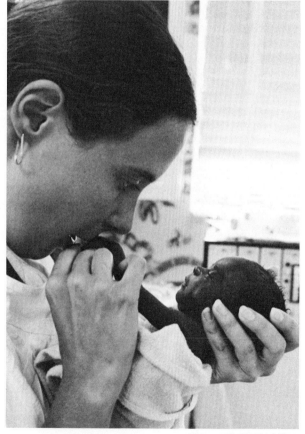

Photo credit: March of Dimes

Premature birth and low birthweight have potentially broad effects on mental health functioning.

usual degree of activity and stimulating behaviors (80,130,145,179,180,181,182). This imbalance frequently results in a vicious cycle, as increased activity on the part of the mother leads to less infant responsiveness, and this, in turn, results in more active maternal behavior. In general, preterm infant-mother dyads have fewer positive interactions than their full-term counterparts, and this difference may increase over the first year of life (130). In normal populations, the quality of early social interactions has frequently been associated with both early and late social, emotional, and cognitive competence. Similarly, it has been found that the less optimal social interactions experienced by preterm infants are related to poorer social, emotional, and cognitive functioning in early childhood (46,181,186,642).

The incidence of the most severe problems associated with premature birth—e.g., cerebral palsy, severe mental retardation, brain damage, epilepsy, and vision and hearing defects (99)—has declined over the last few decades because of improved prenatal monitoring and medical technology (see 635). Nevertheless, infants and children born prematurely are found to display poorer outcomes than full-term infants and children on a variety of developmental indices. Preterm infants have been found to perform more poorly than full-term infants on measures of cognitive, language, and motor development in infancy, including an early assessment of IQ known as the Bayley Scales of Infant Development (80,84,130,185, 195). These problems are especially common in preterm infants of very low birthweight (i.e., less than 1,500 grams). Similarly, toddlers and preschoolers born prematurely tend to perform at lower levels than full-term toddlers and children on tests of cognitive competence (184,185,195, 307,607,642). Again, these differences are much more marked for those born at very low birthweights. In addition to exhibiting lowered cognitive competence, preschoolers born prematurely have been found to display more behavioral symptoms suggestive of minimal brain dysfunction (e.g., hyperactivity, distractibility, short attention span, irritability, impulsiveness, specific fears, and unclear speech); less social maturity; and inferior language production (184,185,186,642).

For many children born prematurely, developmental delays shown in infancy and early childhood are mild and decrease with age. Some effects of prematurity, however, do not fully emerge until the school-age years. These effects frequently take the form of specific cognitive deficits in terms of visuomotor and other perceptual-motor skills (100,307,607). Patterns of specific impairment in perceptual-motor functioning (in the context of normal language performance) are suggestive of learning disabilities (607). In general, children born prematurely have been observed to show poorer school performance than other children (124,140,204,273), although recent research suggests that these differences in long-term outcome may be more related to socioeconomic status than to prematurity (138,148).

In samples of abused and neglected infants and children, preterms are frequently overrepresented (34,168,199,355,583). To the extent that preterms are in greater danger of being abused, they are at risk for experiencing cognitive, social, and emotional difficulties associated with maltreatment detailed above. The cause of the relationship between prematurity and maltreatment is unclear. Factors in the infant, the parent, and the environment, as well as the effects of early separation of preterm infants from their parents, have all been suggested as leading to abuse. It seems likely, however, that none of these factors alone explains the link between prematurity and child maltreatment and, instead, that each contributes to produce a cumulative effect (417).

PARENTAL DIVORCE

Parental divorce can have serious consequences for children's mental health and has increasingly been recognized as an important mental health risk factor. The increasing recognition of its effects is not surprising, given recent increases in the numbers of children under 18 who are living in single-parent households, usually as a result of parental separation or divorce. From 1970 to 1981, the percentage of single-parent families in the United States increased from 12 to 20 percent of households (652). Furthermore, recent estimates suggest that nearly half of the children born in the 1970s and 1980s will spend a portion of their childhood living in a single-parent home (236).

The initial period following separation or divorce is one of severe stress and disorganization for the entire family. During this time, children often exhibit a variety of behavior problems, including oppositional, aggressive behavior (291, 292,293); and depressive reactions and developmental delays (676,677,678,679,680). These problems often occur in children who have had no prior history of psychological difficulty or treatment. Moreover, the problems extend into many parts of children's lives—family relationships, school functioning and academic performance, and relationships with friends. Children from divorced families are more likely than intact-family children to have been referred for psychological treatment (28,265). In addition, children from divorced families have been found to score significantly lower on IQ tests (292), evidence poorer work styles (288), and demonstrate generally lower academic and classroom competence (265).

Many studies report that the various behavior problems exhibited by children immediately after divorce tend to abate without treatment in the 2 years following divorce, especially among girls (294). However, this outcome varies and seems to be related to several mediating variables such as the amount of parental conflict after the divorce. One recent study, using a large, randomly selected sample of children, found that the effects of divorce did not evaporate after 1 to 2 years (266). When compared with intact-family children, children from divorced households (particularly boys) were found to experience a variety of academic, social, mental health, and physical health problems even 5 to 6 years after divorce.

Factors that can either accentuate or ameliorate the negative effects of divorce include the child's relationship with the noncustodial parent, parent adjustment, parents' postdivorce relationship, the child's predivorce adjustment and temperament, the sex and age of the child, and extrafamilial support systems (28). Research varies in the degree to which it has successfully separated the impact of divorce from the impact of other mediating variables (28,169,265,294,370).

MAJOR PHYSICAL ILLNESS

As a result of improvements in the quality of medical treatment, many more children with major chronic illnesses are surviving today who in the past would have died. Although not strictly environmental factors, major physical illnesses are stressful experiences that affect mental health. Chronic diseases that children are now living with and that have demonstrated effects on mental health include cancer (364), cystic fibrosis (151), and chronic renal failure (705). Burn or accident victims and children with congenital abnormalities are also afflicted with mental health problems. Chronic medical conditions that lead to relatively little physical disability, such as epilepsy and diabetes, are also of concern in this context, because these chronic conditions can frequently have greater emotional consequences than conditions which are medically more threatening.

In recent years, it has been recognized that the experience of a major or chronic illness involves complicated psychological and social stresses. Several surveys have found that chronically ill children are at greater risk for developing behavioral or emotional problems than are healthy children (74,425,511,593), although such effects have not been found for all categories of chronic disease (155,633).

The diagnosis of a serious childhood illness can have devastating psychological effects on children and families, even where survival rates and other treatment prospects are good. Children face anxiety over the cause of the illness, its course and prognosis, and the threat it presents to the integrity of their body. They often develop feelings that they are defective and different from their friends, and react with shame and lowered self-esteem. To manage the disturbing feelings, they may deny their illness or develop a sense that parts of their body are alien and separate from themselves, which makes it more difficult to face the reality of their illness (32).

A second source of stress is the effect of the condition itself (705). Experiencing constant pain or severe physical limitations is extremely stressful. Furthermore, a medical condition can limit children's functioning in areas that are especially critical to their stage of development (423,705). Prolonged confinement to bed, for example, interferes with young children's developmental need for movement to explore the world and test their abilities.

An additional source of stress faced by chronically ill children is the difficulty of undergoing diagnosis and treatment. Many techniques used to diagnose and treat illness are uncomfortable, painful, immobilizing, or defacing. Needles to draw blood, biopsies, radioisotopic preparations, and other diagnostic procedures are often more frightening and painful to children than the slow course of a disease. Many treatments of severe diseases (e.g., chemotherapy or radiation therapy) have painful and debilitating side effects. Treatments such as dialysis, which must be continued indefinitely, place enormous psychological demands on children. Furthermore, treatment often forces children to spend long periods of time in a hospital, separated from their parents and friends.

For some children, the greatest stress arises after they return from the hospital. Anxiety remains about the risk that their illness will recur, their body integrity, and their ongoing chances for survival. For children with some conditions, stress is increased because not much is known about their prognosis other than that they are at increased risk for having another episode of the disease (364). Children with major and chronic illnesses may have physical impairment remaining from their illness or from invasive treatment of the illness—either concrete disabilities such as the loss of a limb or more unpredictable problems such as suppression of the immune system. Ongoing treatment regimens, which often involve frequent medication or other treatment, disrupt normal school, peer, and family activities of children. Treatment often continues to be painful or lead to physical changes. Children must rejoin their classroom and peer groups while still coping with the feeling that they are different and,

in many cases, appearing different from other children. The siblings of a sick child may also suffer psychologically because of the illness; they often experience guilt over being well while their brother or sister is ill and jealousy over all the resources and attention devoted to the sick one (152,154, 364). Medical conditions and treatments also interfere directly with children's development, so that they may fall behind in intellectual, emotional, and social development.

The requirements of managing a chronic illness often conflict with the developmental or psychological needs of children. For example, chronic illness forces adolescents to be more dependent on their parents at a time when they need to develop independence. It may lead children to feel both responsible for what happens in the family and guilty over the family's distress. Often the family exacerbates these problems by being overprotective. In general, normal development is made more difficult, because illness necessarily places children in a more dependent, child-like position. Children's prospects for the future can be diminished, partly because their illness impairs their abilities, but also because of prejudice against them in school or at jobs. There is also often prejudice against recovered patients who try to obtain life and health insurance. Several studies have found consequences for adaptation, especially in social relationships, for adults who have had a chronic childhood medical condition (71,237,474). An additional complication is that mental and physical health are closely intertwined; emotional or behavioral problems often exacerbate physical problems. This is true for almost any disease, but especially so for conditions such as asthma in which emotional arousal can stimulate physical symptoms.

Success in coping with a chronic medical condition seems to be related to such factors as the specific course of the medical illness (when it occurs in life, how long it lasts, number of relapses, etc.) and the ability of the family, physician, and others to be supportive (364).

CONCLUSION

A number of biological and psychosocial factors can pose risks to children's mental health. This chapter has examined a number of the more severe environmental risk factors for children—poverty, minority ethnic status, parental psychopathology, physical or other maltreatment, a teenage parent, premature birth and low birthweight, parental divorce, and serious childhood illness. The evidence on many of these factors and their direct relation to children's mental health problems is sometimes unclear, primarily because children exposed to one risk factor may be exposed to others as well.

Consideration of environmental risk factors is important to an examination of children's mental health problems and services. As is acknowledged in diagnostic manuals such as DSM-III, knowledge of a child's physical health status and psychosocial environment is important to developing an effective mental health treatment plan. For policy purposes, it can be important to know that children's mental health problems are not limited to mental disorders, and that it may be possible to prevent development of some mental health problems by reducing certain risk factors (e.g., poverty) and ameliorating the effects of others.

Part III: Services

Chapter 5
Therapies

Therapies

INTRODUCTION

The specific techniques used to treat children with mental health problems vary depending on the nature and severity of a child's problems, the orientation of mental health professionals, and the resources available to finance and house treatment services. Although some treatment methods have been devised especially for children, most are adaptations of procedures used with adults.

This chapter describes the principal treatment methods currently used with children by mental health professionals:

- individual therapy,
- group and family therapy,
- milieu therapy,
- crisis intervention, and
- psychopharmacological (drug) therapy.

In practice, most of these techniques are used in combination with one another.

INDIVIDUAL THERAPY

The paradigm for mental health treatment has traditionally been individual therapy—the one-on-one encounter of a therapist and a patient. Over the past 50 years, there have developed a large number of individually based therapies based on theories as disparate as psychoanalysis and operant conditioning. Each theory has spawned various approaches to individual therapy that have been adapted for use with children.

Three broad categories of treatment approaches used with individual children are described below:

1. *psychodynamic therapy*, which focuses on the development of insight;
2. *behavioral therapy*, which is based on behavioral learning theories and relies on positive and negative reinforcements to create changes in behavior; and
3. *cognitive therapy*, which is based on cognitive learning theories and trains individuals to use new patterns of thinking.

Each of these approaches, though developed to deal with individual patients, can also be used as part of group and family therapy. Furthermore, although psychodynamic, behavioral, and cognitive therapy are based on distinct theories, in practice, many clinicians use an eclectic therapeutic approach.

Psychodynamic Therapy

All forms of therapy for children involve bringing about changes in their cognitions, emotions, and behavior (260). What distinguishes psychodynamic approaches is their emphasis on cognitions and emotions and the concomitant idea that changes in these two realms will be followed by changes in behavior. When psychodynamic approaches are used with children, they often involve elements that are usually not emphasized with adults and that blur distinctions between psychodynamic and other therapeutic approaches with children. These include clarification of conscious feelings and thoughts and aid in the development of alternative problem-solving and coping strategies. The accentuation of these techniques in work with children reflects children's early stage of cognitive and psychosocial development.

Psychodynamic therapy with children is usually accompanied by other interventions. Most often it is accompanied by therapy with the child's parents. The involvement of individuals in the child's environment reflects the fact that children are more dependent than adults and less able to change their environmental conditions.

Psychodynamic child therapy requires considerable resources. A highly trained clinician must provide the therapy, several individuals in the child's environment need to be involved, and frequent therapy sessions may be needed. Psychodynamic child therapy usually involves once- or twice-weekly meetings between therapist and child. There is no predetermined length of treatment, and treatment can last from a few weeks to a few years (9). Because of the resources needed, it is probably more typical that individual therapy with children is psychodynamically informed rather than a pure instance of the psychodynamic model.

A number of mechanisms are thought to account for therapeutic change in psychodynamic child therapy. An emphasis on one mechanism or another may depend on a child's age, the child's relevant strengths and weaknesses, and the severity of the child's problem (207).

Emotional expression by the child and the labeling of emotions by the therapist are primary mechanisms in psychodynamic therapy. The expression of feelings is thought to aid the child by providing him or her with an opportunity for catharsis. The labeling of feelings by the therapist is believed to enable the child to place the feelings in context, thereby reducing his or her sense of being overwhelmed. The therapist's intervention is also thought to help the child understand the connections between thoughts, feelings, and behaviors. The goal is to replace the acting-out of conflicts with feeling, thinking, and verbalization.

Psychodynamic therapy is also hypothesized to aid in the development of ego structure (i.e., a sense of self), which is particularly important for children whose problems began early and who lack self-esteem and impulse control (361). In addition, psychodynamic therapy can provide a child with a "corrective emotional experience." This occurs because the child's usual expectations (e.g., rejection or punishment) are not met, and eventually the "automatic" connections between feelings (e.g., between anger and guilt) no longer occur. Finally, psychodynamic therapy is believed to produce change because it instills hope in the child and fosters the belief that the important people in his or her life are caring and concerned.

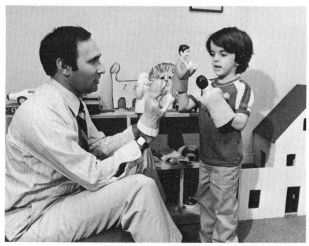

Photo credit: Charter Colonial

In play therapy, problems are approached through games in order to put children at ease.

Despite a well-described theory of the mechanisms of psychodynamic therapy, there are few empirical data to guide decisions about which mechanisms should be emphasized in the treatment of specific problems and particular types of children. Substantial clinical literature suggests that an insight-oriented approach that focuses on widening children's understanding is most applicable for children with relatively good functioning and circumscribed internal conflicts. Children with major developmental problems and limited introspective abilities are probably better served with an approach that stresses problem-solving skills (207,272,481,537).

Psychodynamic therapy is contraindicated in situations in which the parents are unwilling to support the treatment and situations in which the problem is best addressed by altering a child's environment (via the family or school). It is also contraindicated for children who do not have the ability to form a working relationship with a therapist (274).

Behavioral Therapy

Behavioral therapy was developed more recently than psychodynamic therapy, but it is more widely applied in treating children (553). Behavioral therapy assumes that a child learns persistent pathological behavior from his or her experience with the social environment. Therapists using behavioral techniques systematically analyze the child's problem and environment and identify the specific behaviors to be modified. As part of the assessment, frequency counts of maladaptive behaviors may be carefully collected, along with data on the situation within which the maladaptive behavior occurs. Then specific behavioral techniques are applied in an effort to change specific problem behaviors.

Models of Learning on Which Behavioral Therapies Are Based

Several models of learning underlie behavioral therapy methods. The most commonly applied model is *operant conditioning*. This model assumes that learning results from the consequences of behavior (611). Behavior that leads to rewarding consequences is said to be positively reinforced and, as a consequence, is presumed to increase, while behavior that leads to unrewarding or punishing consequences is presumed to decrease. In behavioral therapy based on operant conditioning, adaptive behavior is explicitly rewarded, while maladaptive behavior is either explicitly not rewarded, leads to a delay in reward, or is punished. Thus, for example, children who have problems with aggression and who learn to interact appropriately with classmates may receive special rewards. Some residential treatment settings use "token economies" in which children "earn" tokens that are redeemable for privileges.

A second model for behavioral therapy is *reciprocal inhibition* (716). This model holds that children "learn" an inappropriate, anxious reaction (e.g., a phobia) to an aspect of the environment. Behavioral therapy based on the reciprocal inhibition model usually involves training patients in systematic desensitization—i.e., substituting relaxation or other appropriate behaviors to break the patient's association between a feared object and an inappropriate reaction (37).

A third paradigm, *social modeling or observational learning* (37), is an elaboration of operant conditioning (252). According to this paradigm, an individual learns new behavior by observing another person successfully carrying out the new behavior and being rewarded for it. For example,

observing another child approach a dog could be used to help a child patient overcome a dog phobia.

Applications of Behavioral Therapies

Behavioral therapies are applied in the treatment of children with specific intellectual and developmental disorders, behavior disorders, emotional disorders, and psychophysiological disorders.

Intellectual and Developmental Disorders.—In the case of mental retardation or pervasive development disorders (PDDs), behavioral therapy is not intended as a "cure." It has been used, however, as a major tool for training severely disturbed children to communicate with others and to develop self-care skills (252). Children are trained to use language (305), to develop household skills like telling time and counting change, and to develop social and educational skills. Behavioral methods are sometimes prescribed as specific, intensive, time-limited procedures, but more often they are integrated into a treatment setting's program. For example, meals can be used as part of a behavioral treatment program to teach children to make requests (252). Operant conditioning relying on positive reinforcement has been the mainstay of this training.

Behavioral therapy has often been used in seeking to limit tantrums, self-mutilation, and other self-destructive behaviors in children with PDDs (410). Punishment is used occasionally (e.g., the use of electric shock to stop head-banging), although considerable public and scientific controversy exists about the side effects and ethics of using punishment with children (641).

Behavior Disorders.—A number of behavioral techniques have been developed for treating children with attention deficit disorder with hyperactivity (ADD-H) (129). The contingency management approach requires that parents and teachers use a structured system of rewards contingent on appropriate, attentive behavior by the children.

Behavioral therapy is frequently used with conduct-disordered children in residential juvenile justice facilities. The focus is on improving delinquent children's social or educational skills, while decreasing delinquent behavior within the residential setting (252). Operant conditioning is the primary technique, and token economies are used frequently, but techniques such as behavioral contracting are also employed (591).

Emotional Disorders.—Behavioral techniques have a long history of use in treating children's phobias—a subset of anxiety disorders. Whether desensitization, modeling, or other techniques are employed, most seek to reduce children's anxiety so that they will approach (physically or symbolically) and eventually confront the feared object. Behavioral techniques have not been extensively developed for treatment of emotional disorders other than anxiety.

Psychophysiological Disorders.—Most psychophysiological symptoms are believed to be amenable to behavioral treatment. Therapists have adapted behavioral techniques such as relaxation training, self-control training, and operant conditioning to teach children with stereotyped movement disorders to have greater control over their bodies.

The use of operant conditioning techniques is especially common with enuretic and encopretic children. One such technique, the bell-and-pad technique, for example, places a special device on an enuretic child's bed that sounds a wake-up alarm on contact with a child's urine, teaching the child to associate sleeping with continence (450). Operant conditioning techniques have also been used to treat patients with eating disorders such as anorexia nervosa.

Parent Training in Behavioral Therapy.—Training parents to use behavioral techniques with their children is increasingly favored and has great potential for expansion (251). The application of behavioral techniques by parents has an inherent logic in that parents are responsible for their children and can be directly involved as soon as a problem is identified. It is also an important approach to consider in light of resource constraints and the desirable policy of providing treatment for disturbed children in the least restrictive environment. For some children, a home environment in which the parents apply behavioral techniques can replace the behaviorally programmed environments of residential treatment settings such as psychiatric hospitals and residential treatment centers (RTCs). For the implementation of many behavioral techniques, fairly little training is needed.

Many parents of severely disturbed children have received training in operant conditioning and other behavioral management techniques used in residential treatment settings (398,585). Parents of children with some of the less severe psychophysiological problems have also received training in behavioral techniques, including for example, the bell-and-pad treatment for enuresis. The most common application of parent training is, by far, to childhood behavior problems. These problems can range from tantrums in a toddler, to disruptive classroom behavior (27), to adolescent delinquency. Parents are also reported to have conducted successful behavioral treatments for school phobia (285) and night-time fears (251, 343).

A frequent combination of behavioral procedures taught to parents includes:

1. providing positive reinforcement for appropriate behaviors (usually in the form of attention or praise);
2. avoiding inadvertent reinforcement (e.g., negative attention) for disruptive behavior that is not severe ("extinction"); and
3. segregating children by themselves for more severe disruptive behavior (554).

The use of behavioral contracts is encouraged in some families with conduct-disordered children (252).

Although the techniques of behavioral therapy are relatively simple, especially compared to those of other individual psychotherapies, the analysis of a child's behavior is usually complex, especially when there are multiple dysfunctions. In addition, designing reinforcement schedules and redesigning a child's environment can be more complex than mere description would suggest.

Parents can learn appropriate behavioral techniques from self-help manuals (487), as well as directly from professionals (429). Self-help manuals vary in their quality and their grounding in empirical evidence (235). Since self-help techniques are largely out of the hands of professionals once the books are written and distributed, little is known about the extent, manner, and effectiveness of their use.

Cognitive Therapy

Clinical and research findings indicate that thinking processes of disturbed children are different from those of other children (399,674). Such findings have led to cognitive treatment modalities that attempt to alter the way disturbed children think about their behavior and their environments. Although the way in which cognitive interventions attempt to change thinking varies greatly, two broad classes of cognitive interventions can be identified. One class of cognitive interventions tries to alter the thinking that takes place during a child's troublesome behavior—e.g., by having impulsive, distractible children verbally describe their actions to themselves as they do them (433). The other class of cognitive interventions tries to influence how children think about themselves and others.

Cognitive interventions are used to help children with many types of problems: behavior, learning, emotional, and social problems. One cognitive method derived from theories about neuropsychological functions (399) trains children to use speech as a tool to slow down and focus their learning and behavior (433). Other cognitive interventions train children in such aspects of learning as the amount of time used to respond to a question (436), the visual scanning of educational material, question-asking strategies (143), and analytic abilities (164). Peers and adults who use effective strategies are often used as models.

For emotionally disordered children with phobias, therapists have used behavioral models combined with cognitive training to demonstrate that a feared object or situation can be confronted (351). In addition, various cognitively based training programs have been used to teach emotionally disordered children to solve interpersonal problems more effectively. Other cognitive training programs aim to improve young people's ability to understand and think through social situations (their "social cognition") (643). Such cognitive training may include procedures that teach children the consequences of their behavior for others (621), or train them to take the perspective of others—and to know thereby what behavior would be best in the relationship (643). There may be a significant educational component to these cognitive interventions. For example, some learning groups offer children concrete information about how to improve their social skills (376). Some cognitively based training has focused on training delinquent adolescents the skills necessary to manage group living or a job interview (574).

Cognitive methods are also used with families of disturbed children. For example, some therapists have taught social problem-solving skills to families, especially families of behavior-disordered children (16,347).

In summary, cognitive therapeutic interventions have wide applicability. Cognitive approaches are incorporated in many therapies, and although cognitive approaches require trained mental health professionals, they can be adapted in many settings.

GROUP AND FAMILY THERAPY

Group and family therapeutic approaches are rooted, in part, in theories of individual behavior. They are also based on distinct theories of peer and family relations. Because of the importance of peers and family members or other adults in a child's life, group and family therapy are often used to treat children with mental health problems. The purpose of group therapy is not simply to reduce the cost of treatment by providing treatment to several children simultaneously.

Rather, the goal is to treat aspects of a child's problem which involve interaction with peers and significant adults.

Group Therapy

Although group therapy incorporates elements of other treatments, it is nevertheless a distinct treatment modality. The effectiveness of group therapy is thought to arise from interpersonal processes within the therapeutic group (722). Therapeutic groups are believed to develop an indigenous "culture" (507) and to allow individuals to develop new ways of relating. The strengths of one child become a model for other children, while the entire group can help an individual child address a weakness (230).

The therapist's task in group therapy is to help the group develop helping capacities and to perform organizing and caretaking functions within the group (582). Children in group psychotherapy are a heterogeneous population, and psychotherapy groups are not usually targeted to a particular disorder; most groups aim to address problems in relationships and identity that cut across disorders. Group therapy is thought to be particularly useful for children experiencing difficulties in peer relationships.

Group psychotherapy for children is adapted to the developmental level of the group. Therapy groups for young children are usually organized around group play and activity-oriented social behavior, while adolescent therapy groups rely more heavily on discussion. Particularly for adolescents, the structure of group therapy depends on the level of social relationships among group members.

Group therapy is not always conducted by group therapy specialists. It is sometimes provided by therapists of various orientations (e.g., behavioral and cognitive). Therapists who do not specialize in group therapy typically consider the dynamics of the group less central than other processes. For example, a behavioral therapist may intend group therapy primarily to provide mutual reinforcement for improved behavior or peer modeling (342). Group psychotherapy is often provided as an adjunct to other modalities, particularly individual psychotherapy or family therapy.

Family Therapy

Although most child therapists point to the importance of the family in understanding and treating children, family therapists are distinguished by their unique way of reconceptualizing a set of symptoms. For family therapists, problems do not lie within the child (as suggested by traditional psychiatric diagnosis), but are manifestations of disturbed interactions within a family. A child's symptom is viewed as an indicator of larger family problems and as a response that serves a function for the entire family. Thus, for example, a child's symptom can deflect attention away from more fundamental difficulties such as strife in the parents' relationship (402,442). Because of its functional and protective role, the symptom is reinforcing to the family, and families are psychologically invested in maintaining it. Although family therapy does not necessarily involve the presence of every family member at each session (67), family therapists believe that a child cannot change if the family does not change as well (203,442).

Several models have evolved within family therapy, and each offers different techniques for intervening to produce change. Zimmerman and Sims (736) describe three models: dynamic, systems, and behavioral.

Dynamic models for family therapy are characterized by their reliance on insight as the main method of producing change. Frequently, the focus of insight is on pathological patterns of functioning that are carried from the parents' own past into the present family situation. These patterns may involve conflicts over autonomy and dependency (704), developmental failures that have occurred over generations and are being "projected" onto a child in the current family (612), or situations in which a child's symptom represents an "invisible loyalty" to transgenerational themes (65). Insight into the way in which patterns from the past affect the present is believed to produce growth in all family members, allowing the child to give up the symptomatic behavior.

Systems models for family therapy encompass a diverse group of theorists and techniques. One such model is structural family therapy, an approach most closely associated with Minuchin (443,445). Structural family therapy is aimed at changing the family's psychosocial organization with the expectation that this will produce a change in the experiences of individual members. Family structure, according to Minuchin, is the "invisible set of functional demands that organizes the way in which family members interact" (442). Aspects of family structure that maintain or are the result of dysfunction include family boundaries, alignments, and the balance of power. For example, Minuchin (442) notes that families with an anorectic child are frequently characterized by enmeshed relationships, restrictions on individual autonomy, and lack of conflict resolution. Therapy involves firming up the boundaries between the parental and child subsystems, breaking the facade of mutual agreement between the spouses, and helping them to negotiate conflict. This approach does not preclude separate medical attention for the anorectic child. It does, however, propose that the family, rather than the child, is the matrix within which change must occur.

A related systems model is strategic family therapy (171,172,269,270,684). Strategic family therapists accept the idea that an individual's symptom serves the function of stabilizing and maintaining a balance in the family system. Their approach in therapy, however, is to focus largely on the symptom itself. Specific techniques are used to reveal the changeability of the symptom and to make the previously covert functions and control of the symptom more overt and obvious to all family members. Strategic family therapy does not rely on insight to produce change, and the course of treatment is frequently brief (736).

A third model of family therapy is behavioral family treatment developed by Patterson (487, 490,497). Designed for use with families of conduct-disordered children, Patterson's approach is based on the observation that parents of these children tend to reinforce the occurrence of aggressive behavior and discourage the occurrence of prosocial behaviors (491,492). Parents are trained in the techniques of social-learning-based child management. Through exposure to programmed texts and participation in a parent training group, parents are taught to define, track, and record both deviant and prosocial behaviors in their children and to devise behavioral contracts which specify the consequences of specific behaviors at home.

MILIEU THERAPY

Milieu therapy involves utilizing daily living in a therapeutic setting to teach patients social and educational skills, to explore patients' emotional life and patterns in relating to others, and to provide patients with ongoing support.

The setting in which milieu therapy is provided is either a hospital, an RTC, or a day treatment center. Every aspect of daily life in this setting is shaped to contribute to a child's recovery. Such disparate areas of life as a child's evening routine or how he or she reacts to conflict with another child become opportunities for professional and other staff to intervene and help a child learn more adaptive behavior.

Interventions in milieu therapy can be as prosaic as teaching children to replace rough physical contact with a special handshake or as profound as pointing out a parallel between children's reaction to the staff and their relationship to their family (639). In many therapeutic milieus, the intensive therapeutic relationships that develop with several different staff are thought to give children a chance to re-create and then work out a number of interpersonal difficulties. Behavioral programs are often used as the basis of milieu therapy.

Milieu treatment also includes the group programs used to meet some of the children's needs for education, recreation, and a sense of community. For example, community meetings are held to review events within the hospital and explore their relationship to patients' difficulties. Groups led by professional staff in art therapy, music therapy, and recreation may allow patients to express feelings about their predicament and, at the same time, learn better ways to adapt.

CRISIS INTERVENTION

Crisis intervention is an outpatient treatment based on clinical and other evidence that a major upheaval in a child's life, such as the loss of a family member, can pose an acute threat to the child's mental health (388). Unlike several other approaches, crisis intervention programs often intervene within children's homes. Crisis intervention is sometimes used as an alternative to hospitalization for acute mental health problems. The major goal is to help children and families return to their previous level of functioning. Crisis intervention is usually completed within 6 weeks and often within days (388), but it is often followed by other outpatient treatment.

Crisis intervention techniques emphasize practical steps to defuse threatening situations and to provide family members with coping resources. Specific contracts and emergency plans, for example, are made with family members to lower the level of tension. Suicide prevention is a focus of intervention when necessary, and crisis intervention services are typically offered intensively on an as-needed, off-hours basis. Often, a crisis intervention specialist arranges for additional emergency services, such as emergency caretaking for children to relieve some of the stress on an acutely disturbed parent.

Crisis intervention with children necessarily involves the family; a tenet of the approach is that parents must be helped to develop coping skills necessary to manage in a crisis. The Homebuilders program exemplifies a crisis intervention model that works within children's homes (350). Homebuilders staff begin by uncovering the nature of the family crisis from all viewpoints, defusing tension by letting family members vent their frustrations and concern, and helping the family develop alternative behavioral, cognitive, and emotional means to deal with the critical problem. After the initial intervention(s), contact is maintained until clients are referred to and then receive continuing services.

PSYCHOPHARMACOLOGICAL (DRUG) THERAPY

Psychoactive medication is a small but growing modality of treatment for children's mental health disorders. Although widely used with adults, psychoactive medication has only recently been regularly prescribed for children.

The range of children's mental health problems for which drugs have been prescribed has increased over the last decade. Yet psychopharmacological treatment is not regarded as a panacea for the treatment of any disorder, and there appears to be consensus on the necessity of combining drugs with other treatments.

Stimulants

ADD is one of the few childhood syndromes commonly treated with drugs. The drugs used usually are stimulants, including methylphenidate (Ritalin®) and dextroamphetamine (Dexedrine®). Even though ADD children are generally overactive, stimulant drugs act to increase their attention span. The mechanism underlying the effects of stimulant drugs is not well understood; the best understanding is that such drugs stimulate areas of the brain responsible for maintaining arousal and focusing on specific functions (121). Drug treatment alone is rarely sufficient, and psychological interventions with the child, family, and/or his school environment are usually combined with medication (577).

Neuroleptics

Some children with severely disabling disorders —autism, brain injury, mental retardation— exhibit behaviors that are dangerous to themselves or others. They may, for example, hit other children or destroy furniture when they become excited. Some may develop disabling preoccupations or harmful delusional ideas. Usually, attempts will be made to control their behavior without the use of medication, but in some cases, neuroleptics—also known as antipsychotic medication—will be used.

Neuroleptics may significantly reduce hyperactivity, aggressiveness, and agitation in severely impaired children (89). It should be noted, however, that neuroleptic medication is used not as a treatment to reverse severe disorders, but rather as a means of reducing troublesome symptoms associated with a disorder. Trifluoperazine (Stelazine®) and haloperidol (Haldol®) appear to be the two neuroleptics of choice (89) for such applications, partly because they have fewer sedative effects than other neuroleptics. Recent research (89) has demonstrated that haloperidol reduces stereotyped movements, hyperactivity, deficits in attention, and difficult behaviors in autistic children, and can also be associated with an increase in intellectual functioning. Neuroleptics have little or no direct effect on symptoms such as difficulties in relating to others, although they may have an indirect effect on social functioning by reducing symptoms like agitation. Typically, neuroleptics are used as adjuncts to intensive psychotherapy and other treatments (89).

One concern about most neuroleptics is their sedative effect. Neuroleptics sometimes affect cognitive functions necessary for relating to others,

for learning, and for carrying on daily life—all functions that clinicians aim to increase in severely disabled children. Major tranquilizers can also reduce a child's motivation. Furthermore, the side effects of tranquilizers can be very uncomfortable and sometimes are a source of impairment. Possible side effects include a continuously dry mouth, tremors, and cardiovascular changes. With prolonged use, antipsychotic medications can lead to tardive dyskinesia—an often irreversible movement disorder characterized by uncontrollable repetitive movements of the tongue, lips, head, or neck.

Antidepressants

Antidepressant treatment of childhood depression began in the 1960s (333), but it has not received widespread clinical application. With recent increased interest in childhood depression, research is being conducted on the use of antidepressant medication, especially the tricyclic antidepressants widely used with adults. Drugs have also been used to treat some specific childhood anxiety disorders, although most of these disorders are considered best treated psychologically rather than with drugs (121).

CONCLUSION

The mental health treatments outlined in this chapter are based on diverse theories of children's actions, reactions, and mental disturbances. Some mental health treatments used for children have been developed in response to particular childhood problems, but the majority are adaptations of treatments used for adults and based on general theories of behavior. There is substantial var-

iation in treatment practice based on differing theoretical orientation. Analyzing treatments in terms of their psychodynamic, behavioral, and cognitive assumptions is useful in understanding how treatment decisions are made, although in practice, a number of approaches may be used. The effectiveness of mental health treatments used with children is considered in chapter 8.

Chapter 6
Treatment Settings

Treatment Settings

INTRODUCTION

The settings in which mental health treatment for children is provided greatly influence the intensity of the treatment, the resources required, and the treatment experience of children and their families. This chapter describes treatment settings in the mental health service system: hospitals, residential treatment centers (RTCs), day treatment programs, and outpatient settings such as community mental health centers (CMHCs). Mental health services in non-mental-health settings, preventive services, and the integration of mental health and other services are described in chapter 7.

Following Wilson and Lyman (709), mental health settings can be conceptualized as forming a continuum from most to least intensive. At one end of the continuum is inpatient hospital treatment, which involves 24-hour-a-day care, often for extended periods of time. At the other end of the continuum is outpatient treatment which may involve only 1 or 2 hours a week, or less, sometimes for only a few weeks.

More intensive mental health treatment settings are designed to treat children with more severe problems. Such problems can be either acute, such as suicidal behavior, or chronic, such as infantile autism. In many cases, factors other than the severity of a child's mental problem may indicate the selection of a relatively intensive setting. More intensive settings may be chosen, for example, when children's support systems are insufficient, their home environment is deleterious, or other treatment resources are lacking (457). More intensive settings are also chosen when children may be dangerous to themselves or others.

Intensive mental health treatment settings tend to be restrictive, and this fact necessitates special considerations. Federal legislation such as the Education for All Handicapped Children Act (Public Law 94-142) and judicial decisions such as *Willie M.* v. *Hunt* (see 50) have codified the principle that children should receive appropriate services in the "least restrictive setting" possible. No precise legal meaning of least restrictive setting is available (353), however, and available research does not allow a systematic evaluation of whether the principle is applied appropriately. Consequently, which mental health treatment setting offers appropriate care while still being least restrictive is a matter of clinical judgment influenced by the availability of resources. When optimal or even adequate treatment settings are not available or accessible, the quality of care or the principle of providing care in the least restrictive setting, or both, have to be compromised. Details on trends in the availability and utilization of mental health treatment facilities are provided in chapter 2.

PSYCHIATRIC HOSPITALIZATION

The most intensive and restrictive type of children's mental health treatment is psychiatric hospitalization. Children's psychiatric hospitalization takes place in various types of facilities—in freestanding psychiatric hospitals for people of all ages (both State and county mental hospitals and private psychiatric hospitals), separate children's hospitals or units, chemical dependency units, and, most frequently, in psychiatric units of general hospitals.

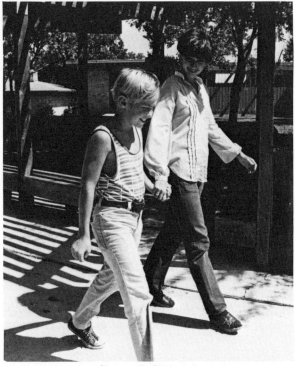

Private psychiatric hospitals generally offer more treatment by psychiatrists than do other mental health settings.

Psychiatric hospitals—regardless of whether they are public or private—are medical facilities that must be licensed as hospitals according to State law (531). Many of these institutions are also accredited as hospitals by the Joint Commission on the Accreditation of Hospitals.

Psychiatric hospitals place disturbed children in an entirely new environment. For the period of a child's institutionalization, the hospital must provide not only for the child's psychiatric care, but also for his or her food, lodging, medical care, recreational needs and, in some cases, education. A host of interventions are used by treatment staff, depending on the hospital. Most hospitals offer individual psychotherapy, family therapy, and group therapy. In addition, medication is used as deemed appropriate. Milieu therapy is central to most psychiatric hospitals, since the 24-hour-a-day environment allows staff to structure the daily life of the ward (activities, interactions

with patients and staff, etc.) to help patients obtain emotional support, learn more adaptive behaviors, and so forth. Many hospital environments also incorporate behavioral interventions.

State and County Mental Hospitals

States and counties provide inpatient psychiatric care to children as part of the public mental health care system, so a substantial number of children's psychiatric beds are in public psychiatric hospitals. States and counties in which it has been recognized that children should be treated differently from adults have begun to open up separate psychiatric hospital programs solely for children. In 1983, there were 30 such facilities in the United States (667). Some child psychiatric inpatient units are an organizational component of CMHCs. Care is generally provided on a reduced-fee basis for those who cannot pay the standard charges, and public sources provide most of the revenues for State and county mental hospitals (667).

During the past 20 years, the number of children treated as inpatients in State and county mental hospitals has declined considerably (724; also see ch. 2) as a result of the deinstitutionalization movement (405). In the vast majority of States, the number of psychiatric beds for children is quite small, and public psychiatric units

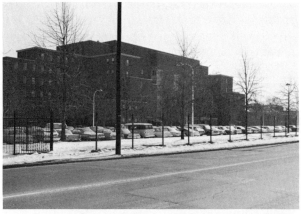

The Dix Building is the child and adolescent treatment facility of St. Elizabeth's Hospital, the public mental hospital in Washington, DC.

are constrained by a lack of fiscal resources. Perhaps as a result, their staffs are less well-trained than the staffs at private facilities (see table 7).

Private Psychiatric Hospitals

Private psychiatric hospitals are owned and administered by various organizations, including private corporations, universities, and religious organizations. The majority are for profit (667). As noted in chapter 2, the mental health services that private hospitals are providing for children are increasing. Typically, private hospitals have more resources to devote to treatment than do public hospitals; consequently, private hospitals tend to provide more hours of ancillary treatment per week per patient, a higher staff-to-patient ratio, and a greater number and level of experience of professional treatment staff.

Private psychiatric hospitalization is the most expensive of the common forms of children's mental health treatment. As of 1986, daily charges were about $375 for a child and about $325 for an adolescent (457). This expense reflects not only the cost of 24-hour institutional care, but also the high cost of medically oriented services (245,587). Reduced-cost or charity treatment in private psychiatric hospitals is provided for only a few cases.

Children's Psychiatric Hospitals and Units

Children's psychiatric hospitals and units can be categorized by the duration of treatment they provide (161). Short-term, acute care psychiatric hospitals or units provide intensive treatment for children in crisis situations when their ability to function deteriorates substantially or they present a danger to themselves or others. Treatment generally lasts no more than 60 days. Short-term psychiatric children's hospital programs offer an alternative environment for disturbed children whose usual environments have rapidly become unable to contain and care for them (60,724). The intent is to treat the most severe and threatening symptoms, help children regain their ability to cope, and prepare them for more long-term, less intensive treatment in another setting.

Intermediate-term psychiatric hospitals for children represent the vast majority of children's inpatient psychiatric facilities. Intermediate-term facilities treat children for periods ranging from about 60 days to about 2 years. Interventions in such facilities are intended to help children make extensive changes in their functioning and often involve significant therapeutic intervention with families.

Table 7.—Distribution of Full-Time Equivalent Staff Positions in Psychiatric Hospitals and Residential Treatment Centers, 1982

Staff discipline	State and county mental hospitals[a]		Private psychiatric hospitals[a]		RTCs for emotionally disturbed children	
	Number	Percent	Number	Percent	Number	Percent
Patient care staff	124,164	65.3%	24,088	63.1%	16,311	72.5%
Professional patient care staff	48,224	25.3	17,408	45.7	10,901	48.5
Psychiatrists	3,866	2.0	1,466	3.8	153	0.7
Other physicians	2,012	1.1	225	0.6	38	0.2
Psychologists (M.A. and above)	3,196	1.7	1,030	2.7	604	2.7
Social workers	6,276	3.3	1,774	4.7	2,100	9.3
Registered nurses	15,613	8.2	5,705	15.0	477	2.1
Other mental health professionals (B.A. and above)	9,179	4.8	5,629	14.8	6,948	30.9
Physical health professionals and assistants	8,082	4.2	1,579	4.1	581	2.6
Other mental health workers (less than B.A.)	75,940	40.0	6,680	17.4	5,410	24.0
Administrative, clerical, and maintenance staff	66,102	34.7	14,057	36.9	6,183	27.5
Total staff	190,266	100%	38,145	100%	22,494	100%

[a]Adult and children's facilities combined.

SOURCE: National Institute of Mental Health; Alcohol, Drug Abuse, and Mental Health Administration; Public Health Service; U.S. Department of Health and Human Services, *Mental Health, United States, 1985*, C.A. Taube and S.A. Barrett (eds.) (Rockville, MD: 1985).

Long-term children's psychiatric hospital units, treating children 2 years or longer, are the least common. Children in long-term facilities are considered chronically disturbed with limited capacity for independence and for maintaining relationships. Many of these children cannot be placed in the community.

Chemical Dependency Units

Chemical dependency units can be either public or private, and can be either freestanding or part of a general hospital. Such units specialize in treating substance abuse and dependence, ranging from alcoholism and alcohol abuse to dependence on use of illicit drugs such as heroin and cocaine. Substance abuse is a DSM-III disorder (see ch. 3), and many private insurers offer reimbursement for its treatment in psychiatric inpatient units. Treatment in some units is especially adapted to the problems of adolescents and/or the types of substances abused by adolescents (709).

General Hospitals With Inpatient Psychiatric Services

General hospitals offer a substantial amount of children's mental health care. Many general hospitals have established separate psychiatric units with treatment programs resembling those of freestanding psychiatric hospitals (60). Psychiatric units in general hospitals tend more often than psychiatric hospitals to focus on short-term, acute care, lasting from a few days to a few weeks or months. In comparison with psychiatric hospitals, psychiatric units of general hospitals also tend to have a somewhat greater proportion of psychiatric patients who have a concomitant medical problem or a psychophysiological disorder, since the general hospital can provide both psychiatric and medical care (60).

Under some conditions, general hospitals admit psychiatric patients to medical wards. In such cases, one or two psychiatric patients may be placed in rooms with medical patients. It is difficult to determine the frequency of such treatment. Critics argue that this form of hospitalization allows assessment of psychiatric problems at best (161) and is probably appropriate only in crisis situations when other resources are not available.

RESIDENTIAL TREATMENT CENTERS

RTCs, as the term is used in this background paper and elsewhere, are 24-hour care settings that provide a mental health treatment program for mentally disturbed children but are not licensed as hospitals (531).

RTCs range from highly structured institutions that follow something resembling a medical model and function somewhat like psychiatric hospitals to less medically oriented institutions that are sometimes hard to distinguish from halfway houses, group homes, and foster care homes (531). In comparison to RTCs, psychiatric hospitals tend to have a greater mix of professionals and greater involvement by psychiatrists and psychiatric nurses (see table 7). Furthermore, psychiatric hospitals may often admit certain children whom RTCs might not admit—in particular, children who are highly aggressive, suicidal, or overtly psychotic (with delusions or hallucinations) (60, 411,724). It is becoming more common for hospitals and RTCs to be operated by the same organization and to exist side by side on the same grounds (see ch. 10)

The size of RTCs, in terms of numbers of patients, ranges from a few children to hundreds. According to 1981 data, about 75 percent of the under-21-year-old patients treated by RTCs are adolescents 12 to 17 years old; approximately 19 percent are 6 to 11 years old; less than 1 percent are 5 years of age or less (724).

The intensity of treatment provided in RTCs ranges from the provision of virtually every service possible to only custodial care. Like psychiatric

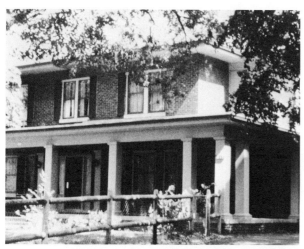

Photo credit: Horizon, a division of Shadow Mountain Institute

RTCs are 24-hour-care settings that provide a mental health treatment program for mentally disturbed children but are not licensed as psychiatric hospitals.

The goal in these RTCs is to enable severely disturbed children to attain the highest level of development possible, to allow these children to eventually return to the community.

One noteworthy model of RTC treatment (also extended to day treatment) is called Project-Re-ED, described originally as a "project for the re-education of emotionally disturbed children" (300). Although Re-ED programs are generally residential, much of their work is based on what Hobbs called "ecological strategies"—changing a child's mental health problem by working both with the child *and* the family and community from which the child comes.

Re-ED programs approach children's mental health problems as the result of unhealthy interaction between children and their environments and intervene accordingly. Approximately one-third of Re-ED staff work full-time with parents, teachers, and other community members to help them change their interactions with the child being treated at Re-ED. Staff may advise parents, for example, on strategies to help their children maintain self-centered, or collaborate with teachers in designing a program for a child who is returning to a school in the community. Almost all children in Re-ED programs return home for weekends to maintain their contact with family and community.

At Re-ED residences, "teacher-counselors" work to bolster children's academic competence and emotional well-being. Academic progress is seen as a key step in reducing mental health problems and promoting the child's return to the community. Re-ED also emphasizes milieu therapy, with one-on-one intervention between staff and child taking place mainly in the context of the milieu, and little or no individual therapy. The positive emotional experiences of daily life at a Re-ED program are thought to form a large part of the treatment.

hospitals, RTCs place disturbed children in an entirely new environment and are responsible for all aspects of care. RTCs employ most of the therapies discussed in chapter 5. Milieu therapy is also central to RTC treatment.

The length of stay in an RTC ranges from days to a year or more. Most RTCs, over 80 percent, treat children for a period ranging from several months to 2 years (724). The goal in these settings is to return children to the community after extensive efforts to increase their level of daily functioning. A smaller percentage of RTCs, less than 15 percent according to Young (724), treat children for more than 2 years on the average. RTCs that provide long-term care primarily serve severely disturbed children (e.g., those with infantile autism, more severe mental retardation, neurological disorders). In these settings, it is recognized that patients will not "recover" from their conditions, nor ever approach normal development.

DAY TREATMENT/PARTIAL HOSPITALIZATION

Some children do not need 24-hour treatment but do require more intensive treatment than 1 or 2 hours a week of therapy. Day treatment often is used as a followup to psychiatric hospitalization or RTC treatment, when a child may no longer need 24-hour care but is not yet ready to cope with a regular classroom. Day treatment programs provide extended treatment, available for a number of hours daily, and can provide a range of therapies that are not available at clinics. Some programs provide treatment to children before or after regular school hours, while other programs provide education to children whose troubles prevent them from attending school.

Some day treatment programs are designed according to an educational model. These programs, sometimes called psychoeducational day treatment programs, operate more like schools than other day treatment centers but incorporate a therapeutic component within the educational program. Their curriculums in many cases are adapted from regular school curriculums, but include special approaches to address the almost universal learning problems of mentally disordered children. Like psychiatric hospitals and RTCs, day treatment centers offer the kind of extensive daily environment in which milieu therapy can be done. Model day treatment programs also include mental health components involving individual therapy, group therapies, family therapy, vocational counseling, and other vocational programs. They also provide other educational and recreational activities designed to further the development of adolescents in a less treatment-oriented fashion.

Partial hospitalization is the use of a psychiatric hospital setting for less than 24-hour-a-day care for given patients. For example, some children might need the treatment offered in the hospital setting during the day but be able to return home in the evening. The treatment program for those children would be identical to the daytime treatment program of the inpatient children. In effect, this is day treatment applied in a psychiatric hospital setting.

OUTPATIENT SETTINGS

Outpatient treatment settings are by far the most prevalent settings used for children's mental health treatment. CMHC outpatient departments, private outpatient clinics, and private mental health practices are described below. Most of the treatment modalities discussed in chapter 5, from individual psychotherapy to group and family therapy, can be provided in these settings.

CMHC Outpatient Departments

Initially established by the Federal Government through the Community Mental Health Centers Act of 1963, CMHCs were intended to provide comprehensive mental health services to all the residents of a catchment area regardless of their ability to pay. The mental health services provided by CMHCs include treatment, prevention, and consultation and education services, but outpatient treatment is by far the most common.

CMHC care is provided to adults (619), but most centers also provide some children's services. Some CMHCs have incorporated previously established child guidance clinics, while others have established new child treatment services. CMHCs use virtually all treatment modalities, including psychodynamic psychotherapy, behavior therapy, cognitive therapy, psychosocial interventions, parent guidance, family therapy, and psychopharmacological (drug) therapy. For the majority of children, more than one modality of treatment is provided simultaneously (363), usually including one or more interventions directly with the child plus work with important adults in the child's life.

Despite the intentions of the 1963 law, a network of CMHCs never developed as a nationwide mental health care system. Furthermore, according to some observers (619), the network that did develop slighted the needs of children for several years. Few CMHCs included children's services when they were established, and in those that did establish child services, the resources available for such services were often too low. The number of staff devoted to children was small, and the level of training of the staff in child mental health was poor (9,11,55,514). The situation improved somewhat in the 1970s; according to a 1981 survey from the National Institute of Mental Health (NIMH), approximately 17 percent of the resources of CMHCs were devoted to children's mental health care (665).

In 1981, direct Federal support for CMHCs was withdrawn. Federal funds began to be provided to CMHCs indirectly via the States through the block grant mechanism (see ch. 10).

Private Outpatient Clinics

In addition to CMHCs, many private clinics provide outpatient treatment to mentally disturbed children. The services that private clinics provide resemble CMHC outpatient services in many ways, although private clinics vary more in size, scope, and treatment philosophy. Unlike most CMHCs, private clinics do not have the responsibility to provide for all the mental health treatment needs of a given community. Many closely adhere to the philosophy of the individuals administering the clinic. Some private clinics are nonprofit and have sliding scales for payment (e.g., Family Service Association centers), while others provide services only at standard fees.

Some clinics were established as child guidance clinics prior to the development of CMHCs and have not been absorbed into CMHCs.

Private Mental Health Practices

Many mental health professionals provide outpatient child mental health care in private practice. The number of children seen by private practitioners is not known, but it is believed to be lower than the need. Private mental health care practitioners include psychiatrists, psychologists, clinical social workers, psychiatric nurses, and mental health counselors who have met State licensing standards. In form and method, private practice resembles outpatient treatment in organizational settings. However, private practitioners generally charge fees affordable only by families with middle incomes and above, and then often only with help from insurance. With widespread availability of health insurance, some private care is accessible to most families, but insurance policies vary greatly in their coverage of outpatient mental health care (374).

CONCLUSION

Mental health treatment settings that provide services to children are diverse, ranging from hospital and RTC settings to day treatment centers to outpatient settings. They can be arranged along a rough continuum according to their intensiveness. Even within a type of setting, settings vary in their form of administration (public versus private), cost, type of children served, duration of treatment, and philosophy of treatment.

The need for availability of a diversity of settings to treat the range of children's mental health problems has been repeatedly emphasized. For example, the President's Commission on Mental Health (514) recommended both an increase in the number of hospital and RTC facilities for seriously disturbed children and an expansion in the availability of community-based mental health care of all types (e.g., hospital, RTC, outpatient) for all children.

One factor contributing to the need for a diversity of mental health treatment settings is the desirability of providing appropriately intensive mental health treatment in the least restrictive setting possible. It is easier to strike a balance between intensiveness and restrictiveness when treatment settings are available that cover the range of these dimensions. For children who need more intensive treatment than can be provided in weekly office visits but who can still live at home, the most appropriate setting—if it is available—may be a day treatment program.

Another factor that underlies the need for multiple mental health treatment settings is the fact that many children, especially those who are severely disturbed, require either concurrent or consecutive treatment from more than one setting. For example, some children who go to an outpatient clinic once a week for psychotherapy to address specific emotional issues might also benefit from participation in day treatment to learn daily living skills. Or children discharged from a psychiatric hospital may live, initially, in a less intensive RTC and later receive psychotherapy as an outpatient in the community.

The variety of mental health treatment settings described in this chapter does not imply that all children have access to the full range of possible settings. Although many different models have been developed, the number of settings available is much more limited. The overall number of mental health treatment facilities is fairly small. Furthermore, access to some settings is limited by cost. Many families cannot afford the costs of treatment in private psychiatric hospitals or RTCs or through private practices. The number of treatment openings for children in public psychiatric hospitals, RTCs, and day treatment centers is severely limited, and the development of child outpatient treatment in CMHCs has not been comprehensive.

Chapter 7

Treatment in Non-Mental-Health Systems, Prevention, and the Integration of Mental Health and Other Services

Treatment in Non-Mental-Health Systems, Prevention, and the Integration of Mental Health and Other Services

INTRODUCTION

Mental health treatment, it is widely agreed, should take place in the context of a child's life. Children are uniquely dependent on their families, schools, and communities, and are continually affected by these influences. Disturbed children are more likely than other children to fail in school, to manifest a variety of medical problems, and to be involved with the criminal justice system. As a result, children's mental health problems are often first identified in settings such as schools, physicians' offices, and juvenile courts. These settings, along with others, provide important mental health treatment sources.

Understanding how treatment services are offered in non-mental-health contexts, such as the educational, health care, welfare, and juvenile justice systems, is essential for developing public policy. The interrelationship between mental health and other service systems provides opportunities to identify children in difficulty, to provide interventions at the site where mental health problems are identified, and to offer programs to prevent mental health problems. Currently, however, there is relatively little integration among mental health and other systems. This chapter considers needs for and provision of mental health services across various non-mental-health systems. It describes a number of programs and projects in the educational system, the health care system, the child welfare system, and the juvenile justice system, along with the development of integrated service systems.

CHILDREN'S MENTAL HEALTH TREATMENT IN NON-MENTAL-HEALTH SYSTEMS

Treatment in the Educational System

The importance of dealing with children's mental health problems in the educational system has long been recognized (see 602). Mental health problems interfere with a child's ability to learn and to manage in the social world of the school. Moreover, mental health problems are likely to have a great effect at school simply because of the number of hours that children spend there and the importance of education to their lives. Many children can receive an adequate education only if their mental health needs have been met.

Schools deal with the mental health needs of children in a variety of ways (157), but the potential of the educational system in meeting children's mental health needs has not been fully realized. A tradition of referring children from schools to mental health treatment settings dates back to the child guidance clinics of the 1920s and 1930s. Some schools have their own mental health professionals, such as school psychologists and social workers, who provide mental health treatment within the school and provide consultation to other school staff (see 372). Other schools rely more heavily on external mental health professionals and a variety of referral resources. A subspecialty of education, special education, was specifically developed to serve the educational needs of children with learning disabilities and psychological and physical handicaps. Because of the difficulties involved in innovation in public schools

(407) and the difficulty of collaboration between the educational system and mental health system (437), mental health interventions in schools have not been widely implemented. Nevertheless, there has been substantial experimentation with such interventions. Experimental programs have provided extra classroom interventions for hyperactive children, learning-disordered children, conduct-disordered children, anxious (withdrawn) children, or heterogeneous groups of disturbed children. These experimental programs in schools have involved various therapeutic approaches. Behavioral interventions have been used extensively since the 1960s, and the use of cognitive interventions such as self-control and social skills training has been increasing. These interventions have been implemented by both teachers and mental health professionals.

The Education for All Handicapped Children Act (Public Law 94-142) requires that an education be provided to all physically and mentally handicapped children. For each handicapped child, the necessary educational and related services to enable the child to obtain an education must also be provided. The law requires the development of an individualized education program that specifies those educational and related services for each child. There has been some dispute over what a "related service" is and whether mental health treatments such as psychotherapy fall within that definition. There is a growing consensus that mental health treatments are related services, and this view has been supported by several court decisions (e.g., *Papacoda* v. *State of Connecticut*, 528 F. Supp. 68 [D. Conn. 1981], *In the matter of the "A" Family*, 602 P. 2d 157 [Mont. 1979]), cited in 358).

Who is to provide and who is to pay for educational and mental health services for disturbed children under Public Law 94-142 has been unclear. In some States, schools themselves offer psychological services, although school personnel providing such services often have less clinical training than out-of-school providers. When mental health services are provided in nonschool settings, it is often unclear whether the responsibility for payment rests with the schools or with

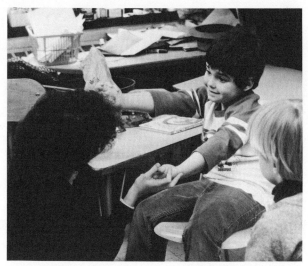

Photo credit: Very Special Arts

In general, mental health professionals believe that the least restrictive setting is most appropriate for treating children. Here, the educational system offers a valuable non-mental-health setting in which to treat children.

the parents. This is especially unclear when the necessary related service is a residential treatment. In 1984, 4 million students aged 3 to 21 received services under Public Law 94-142. The number of handicapped children receiving mental health services is not known.

The Federal contribution to activities mandated by Public Law 94-142 is relatively small: $1.07 billion in fiscal year 1984, 25 percent of which was set aside for administrative and other support services, including "related health services" (657). Essentially, however, services for handicapped children are mandated, but resources are not provided to implement them. It is not known what portion of funds for psychological and mental health were spent for psychological services. A study to assess amounts spent by educational agencies on all related services, including psychological services, is due to be completed in fiscal year 1987 (656). The form that implementation of Public Law 94-142 should take is still being determined in a number of States, and responsibilities across education departments, mental health departments, and other service systems are still being considered.

Treatment in the General Health Care System

Increasing evidence suggests that many children's mental health problems are seen by physicians in the course of delivering primary health care; but surveys differ on the extent to which office-based primary care physicians see and recognize mental health problems in children. In two recent surveys by Goldberg, et al., pediatricians reported that approximately 5 percent of the children they saw had a mental health problem (239, 240). Schurman and colleagues, using data from the National Ambulatory Medical Care Survey, found that about 11 percent of office visits to pediatricians and about 12 percent to family practitioners were by children with psychiatric disorders (588).

In Goldberg, et al.'s investigation, the majority of troubled children visited their physician's office because of a physical complaint, and their mental health problems were uncovered during the course of visits for other problems. Pediatricians often treated the mental health problems themselves, providing supportive counseling, practical advice or, less frequently, medication (239). Approximately 50 percent of the pediatricians in Goldberg, et al.'s samples (239,240) referred troubled children to a mental health professional.

Some observers are concerned about the level of mental health knowledge of many primary care physicians (239,240). Furthermore, although primary care physicians and mental health professionals may see child patients concurrently, their efforts are not always coordinated.

Two options open to many primary health care providers are obtaining mental health training (e.g., 85) and consulting with mental health specialists (543). The logic behind increasing the mental health skills of primary care providers is that they are likely to be the first professionals consulted regarding developmental and psychological problems of young children (504).

In addition to mental health consultation and mental health training for primary care providers, early intervention programs have been developed in primary medical care settings for children suffering from a number of childhood problems (536).

Prevention efforts have been used to help physically ill pediatric patients manage their illnesses without undue mental health consequences (323). Systematic mental health interventions in physical health care settings remain exceptional, however. Only in settings such as health maintenance organizations might mental health referrals and interventions be commonplace.

Evidence for the susceptibility of chronically ill and physically disabled children to mental health problems was noted in chapter 4. The prevalence of mental health problems seen by medical specialists in medical inpatient units is probably high.

Treatment in the Child Welfare System

The child welfare system is involved with a substantial number of children who have serious problems. Child welfare systems intervene in cases of parental abuse and neglect and in other situations in which parental care is lacking (e.g., during a parent's illness).

Treatment Needs for Children in Foster Care

A major form of intervention by child welfare authorities is foster placement. The child welfare system places an estimated 120,000 children per year in some form of foster care, usually within a home or institutional setting (48). There has been little research to ascertain what portion of this population enters foster placement with mental health needs.

Children generally enter the foster care system from family situations with problems including child maltreatment, parental psychopathology, and parental substance abuse—all of which are risk factors for mental health problems (see ch. 4). Only a small percentage of children have been placed in foster care because of their own behavior or disability (108). When placed in foster care, children suffer the trauma of separation from their original families (205). Many children who would be diagnosed as having psychological problems by mental health professionals are not recognized as having such problems by foster care placement agencies and staff (205). For the most part, these children are not placed in environments capable of providing appropriate care for psychological problems (205).

Frank's study of treatment needs for children in foster care found that children involved in long-term foster care typically had severe psychosocial problems (205), both at the point of entry into foster care and 5 years later. Children who were rated at a level of medium to low functioning at entry into foster care slipped significantly to the lower level after the 5-year period. Frank found that 85 percent (composite percentage) of the sample of children in long-term foster care received inadequate treatment (apart from the quality of child care).

Several State studies suggest that the prevalence and severity of emotional disturbance is associated with the number of placements a child has experienced (108). Long-term and repetitive foster care placement, therefore, are likely to represent both sources and symptoms of problems for children with mental health needs. Yet child welfare agencies often have neither the money nor the experienced staff to provide mental health services, and coordination between welfare and mental health agencies is rare (358).

Alternatives to the usual pattern of foster placements are discussed below. These alternatives are therapeutic foster care, respite care, and care in group homes. Efforts to prevent the need for foster placement by enhancing parents' abilities to care for their children are discussed later in this chapter.

Therapeutic Foster Care

Mentally disturbed children who might otherwise be referred to psychiatric hospitals or residential treatment centers (RTCs) are sometimes placed in alternative family settings (83). Although separating a child from his or her parents is a significant intervention, therapeutic foster care is considered less intensive than treatment in a psychiatric hospital or RTC.

Well-run therapeutic foster care programs carefully select foster parents to take disturbed children into their homes for a finite period of time. These foster parents are generally expected to provide some therapeutic work and are typically paid more than other foster parents. Such parents, who

vary in their experience with mental health treatment, undergo training prior to therapeutic foster care placement. Professionals involved with foster care programs supervise and support the foster parents, arrange for other care needs of the disturbed children in foster care, and provide emergency professional care for foster children when needed.

The range of the intensiveness of treatment within therapeutic foster care programs is substantial, and the more intensive levels require more treatment-specific training, greater involvement of foster parents, and greater availability of adjunct services. In many States, different levels of therapeutic foster care are available to cover a range of impairment in children.

Children in therapeutic foster care usually receive mental health treatment beyond therapeutic foster care. The nature of this other treatment depends on the particular child's needs and the availability of local resources. Thus, for example, one child in therapeutic foster care may receive outpatient psychotherapy, while another may attend a day treatment program.

Respite Care

Respite care, a service related to foster care, involves placing children in homes with caring adults as an emergency intervention. Respite care provides children in need with a temporary protected environment. Such care may be necessary because of a crisis such as the emotional breakdown of parents or escalating conflict between children and other family members. Shelter from a crisis may be provided for several days or up to several weeks, until the child can return home or be placed in another appropriate setting.

Group Home Care

Group home care is similar to therapeutic foster care, except that a number of children (usually 10 to 12) are placed in a home at one time (709). Group homes are typically administered by social service agencies, which employ staff to live in the home or work there in shifts. Group homes usually have a somewhat more structured treatment program than therapeutic foster homes. Placement in group homes can last anywhere from

1 month to several years, and commonly includes concurrent treatment in a mental health setting.

Treatment in the Juvenile Justice System

The juvenile justice system is a potentially major site for provision of mental health care to disturbed children and adolescents. By DSM-III criteria (see ch. 3), juvenile offenders with a history of behaviors such as fighting, stealing, lying, and running away from home would be diagnosed as having a conduct disorder. Often, however, the mental disorders of juvenile offenders are not formally diagnosed, and the number of juveniles who have mental disorders in addition to criminal or status offenses (offenses that are criminal only because the offender is a juvenile, e.g., truancy, running away from home) is not actually known.

The proportion of children and adolescents in the juvenile justice system who are regarded as mentally disordered or as having mental health problems obviously depends on what criteria are used to define mental disorders and mental health problems (601,723). Whether a child's problems are dealt with in the mental health system or in the juvenile justice system often appears to depend less on characteristics of the child than on how a particular behavior is defined (i.e., as a symptom or as a violation of the law) and on the system within a State or region for assigning service responsibility.

Coordinated interventions in which both the mental health and the juvenile justice system are involved are rare (395). Mental health agencies are often reluctant or unable to take responsibility for intervention with juvenile offenders because of the danger and disruptiveness these children and adolescents present, and the juvenile justice system is often unable to treat the mental health problems of these youths. Many mentally disordered children have contact with both the mental health and juvenile justice systems, often moving back and forth between the systems. Frequently, children who are sent from one system to the other are those for whom original interventions have failed or been exhausted (395,723). The frequent and rapid transferring of these "turn-stile" children (276) sometimes causes problems itself.

There are several models of coordinated mental health and juvenile justice interventions (601). A number of special mental health programs have organizational connections to State and county governments and provide comprehensive services to disturbed juvenile offenders (49,304,395,723). In some instances, States contract with private mental health agencies to provide services to children who come in contact with the juvenile justice system in specific geographic areas (395). Other programs provide mental health consultation directly to juvenile justice facilities (395,601). Case management (discussed below) has been used to resolve some of the problems of trying to serve disturbed children who are wards of the juvenile justice system, but the use of case management in the juvenile justice system is infrequent (49).

PREVENTION OF CHILDREN'S MENTAL HEALTH PROBLEMS

A number of strategies are used to prevent behavioral, social, emotional, and academic difficulties in children. Primary prevention strategies are aimed at reducing the incidence of new cases of mental health problems; secondary prevention efforts are directed at reducing the severity and duration of disorders through early identification, diagnosis, and treatment (see 98). In practice, however, primary and secondary prevention often overlap. The common objective underlying all prevention efforts is to reduce the incidence of mental health problems in the population and to reduce the need for more intensive and costly treatment services such as psychiatric hospitalization or other residential treatment (98).

Primary Prevention

Primary prevention efforts are frequently directed at parents and educators. Sometimes they are aimed at the parents of children who are at high risk. To treat high-risk infants, for example, programs train parents in different techniques for stimulating and giving attention to the infant. Other similar primary prevention interventions have been developed for particular groups (e.g., poor women) and teenage mothers (187,525).

Primary prevention methods have also been devised for the parents whose children are not known to be at high risk. Such methods include training manuals to help instruct parents in child-management techniques (e.g., 40,429,497), educational videotapes for inexperienced mothers (78), and parent education groups such as Parent Effectiveness Training (242,243). Although popular, some of these methods have been criticized for not meeting the needs of low-income families (110).

In school settings, primary prevention efforts include alcohol education programs in elementary schools (380) and mental health consultation services provided to teachers (see 408). Such efforts also include programs aimed at decreasing specific behaviors that are thought to predispose children to later problems in school adjustment. For example, one program employed intensive training in interpersonal, cognitive problem-solving for kindergarten children in the hopes of decreasing inhibited and impulsive behavior and enhancing social problem-solving skills (621).

Head Start and similar preschool child development programs are examples of an ongoing effort at primary prevention. Head Start was established as a national program in 1965 to provide enriched early childhood education for low-income children. Head Start also provides a range of other services, including health, nutrition, and social services. The program emphasizes parent and community involvement in the development and operation of the program, a feature that has proved effective (see ch. 9). However, Head Start has been criticized for devoting few resources and little attention to mental health services (308).

Somewhat different from other primary prevention programs are family support programs. In recent years, the importance of families for children's mental health has been widely acknowledged (290). Although families are often viewed as the primary contributors to mental illness in children, they are increasingly recognized as a

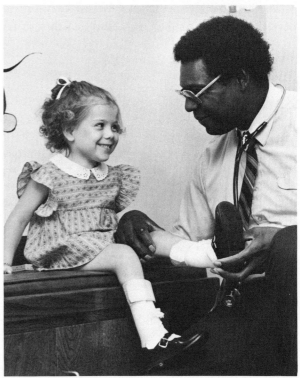

Photo credit: March of Dimes

Physically disabled children may be susceptible to mental health problems.

principal source of mental health and adaptation (693).

The idea of supporting families is not new, but the growth of a family support movement as a distinct and important aspect of children's mental health services is a fairly recent phenomenon (326,693). The family support movement can be said to be integrative in that it focuses on the needs and linkages between children, families, communities, and broader social systems. According to Weiss (693) and others (594), the family support movement evolved in part from early intervention and prevention programs such as Head Start. The finding that the most effective of these programs were those that actively involved parents —and the related idea that children at risk need an intervention approach that encompasses more than educational enrichment—pointed to the family as a necessary focus of intervention.

More recently, the family support movement has gained impetus from research underscoring the importance of quality parent-child interactions in promoting children's social, emotional, and cognitive competence (e.g., 623). The development of family support programs has also been supported by recent trends in the delivery of social services. Such trends include increasing emphasis on the promotion of health and the prevention of illness, the use of self-help and mutual aid groups, and access and coordination of services through information and referral systems (334,693).

Finally, the family support movement is a response to the stresses faced by contemporary American families. Such stresses include demographic trends (e.g., increases in the numbers of single-parent and dual-career households) as well as broad social forces such as unemployment, economic uncertainty, and increased mobility and isolation of families.

The family support movement represents a diverse array of services and programs that share underlying assumptions and conceptual emphases more than a particular format or structure. Family support services range from a center-based program resembling traditional mental health service to practices such as corporate flexitime and daycare.

Family support programs are characterized by their focus on family strengths rather than deficits; their recognition that parents need and want information and support in carrying out their roles; an attempt to empower families and foster self-reliance; and their emphasis on the relationship not only between children and parents, but also between families and the sources of support in their communities.

According to Weiss (693), the dimensions on which family support programs vary include the type of family served (e.g., new families, single-parent families, families with special needs); service delivery mechanisms (e.g., newsletters, home visits, parent groups); program goals (e.g., child abuse prevention, home and school linkages, parent and child education); program settings (e.g., mental health centers, schools, churches, drop-in centers); staff composition (e.g., mental health and health professionals, educators, volunteers); and funding sources (private and public).

Two examples of family support programs are the Yale Child Welfare Research Program (594) and the Family Support Center Program (see 202). The Yale Child Welfare Research Program is different from other programs in that it is university based and includes outcome research as one of its major components. The Yale program is typical of family support interventions, however, in that it employs a multidisciplinary teamwork approach focused on the social and emotional adjustment of all family members. The goal of the Yale program's interventions is to enhance parent's ability to perform their caregiving roles and to solve their own life problems. Interventions are aimed at impoverished families considered at risk by virtue of the chronic stresses and limited resources associated with reduced socioeconomic status. Families receive home visits, pediatric care, daycare, developmental examinations, and psychological services as needed, and services are provided over a 2½-year period for each family. In a recent 10-year followup of the original program participants and an equivalent group of control families, the Yale program's interventions were found to have both positive and long-lasting effects (see ch. 9).

The Family Support Center Program is designed to reduce the incidence of child maltreatment in at-risk families by providing parents with support and guidance in a series of steps that emphasize progressively greater peer support and progressively less staff involvement. As parents advance in the program, they move from receiving direct staff support and consultation, to attending a "family school" with their children, to participating in a neighborhood support group. An evaluation of a Family Support Center Program (25, 202) is discussed in chapter 9.

Secondary Prevention

Secondary prevention efforts for children who have begun to show signs of behavioral difficulties have been implemented in both home and school settings. Some secondary prevention efforts are aimed at training parents to deal directly with their children's problems. In one program (317,318), parents were taught to use behavioral methods to modify a range of behaviors in their preschool children at home (e.g., reducing aggression and tantrums, and increasing eye contact, imitation, and vocalization). This program also involved parents in health-center-based activities in which they observed and were instructed in teaching activities aimed at enhancing their children's prosocial behavior and language skills.

One of the most extensively implemented and well-researched school-based secondary prevention programs is the Primary Mental Health Project (PMHP) of Cowen, et al. (128). This program was developed to remediate children's problems in the primary grades, a goal based on observations that early school problems frequently persist or increase over time and that they lead to more serious mental health problems later in life (126,128). PMHP involves the delivery of individually based, remedial efforts to grade-school children who have been identified as having behavioral and academic difficulties (e.g., acting-out, withdrawal, and learning problems). Teacher aides meet with children on a regular basis during the school year, and individual goals are modified according to the child's changing needs. Additionally, mental health professionals serve as consultants to teachers and other school personnel. The PMHP model has been widely disseminated, and programs have operated in over 200 schools throughout the country (125).

INTEGRATION OF MENTAL HEALTH AND OTHER SERVICES

As described in this chapter, the treatment and prevention of children's mental health problems occurs in a variety of settings—educational and other—outside the mental health care system. In addressing children's needs, therefore, it is important to consider the integration of mental health services with other services. Given the diverse settings in which children's mental health care is provided, it is perhaps not surprising that fragmentation of services is often reported (324,359).

Isaacs (310,311) has reviewed various methods of integrating systems, both at the level of entire systems or programs and at the level of individual children. State departments can cooperate at the administrative level to develop policy decisions together, to initiate programs jointly, or to share management and support services. Service programs can include staff from all systems. At the level of the individual child, agencies can collaborate on most stages of the treatment process, from case finding and evaluation to followup. Although each agency provides specialized services, staff from different services can collaborate in periodic case conferences, case teams, or case consultation.

According to Isaacs (312), a number of principles should undergird the organization of the children's mental health system. One is that children's mental health services should be integrated with services that address a child's physical, mental, social, and intellectual needs while recognizing the developmental stages of the child and the needs of different groups of children and adolescents. Another principle is that services should be coordinated, with a single agency given responsibility for developing and coordinating the system of care at both local and State levels. Yet another important principle is that services should be delivered to the extent possible within the child's normal environment (i.e., home, school, health care setting), and, if such is not possible, within the least restrictive environment. Finally, early identification of problems should be promoted and the system of care should support a child's right to develop in a nurturing environment with positive adult relationships.

One important concept in the integration of children's services is that of the case manager or case advocate (359). A case manager or advocate is an individual or team, usually in the mental health system, who assumes responsibility for ensuring that the appropriate combination of services from all service systems is provided to a client. Case managers are conversant with the laws entitling children to services, such as Public Law 94-142, and ensure their application in individual cases by advocating on the child's behalf in school, in court, or within the mental health treatment program itself (359). They can maintain the push for treatment within systems that are sometimes overwhelmed, disinclined to treat difficult children, and entangled in bureaucratic difficulties (359).

One of the most sophisticated models of case management has been developed by North Carolina. In this model, case managers are responsible for seeing that all facets of a child's evaluation and treatment are carried out. They continually review the treatment plan and monitor its implementation; one of their responsibilities is seeing to it that the disturbed child receives treatment in the least restrictive setting possible (50). In some instances, case managers locate and arrange for services outside the mental health system, such as homemaking systems for beleaguered mothers, that are nonetheless crucial to the stability of a disturbed child's family. In addition, they arrange for the adult service systems to continue care for children in need who are about to turn 18 (50).

At present, the integration of mental health and other children's services is probably more of an ideal than a reality. In a review of State administrative structures for provision of coordinated services, Isaacs (313) concluded that despite a number of models, implementation of coordination plans often depends on the efforts of individual staff members, rather than on established systems and structures. In addition, Isaacs (313) found that even in States attempting coordination between the mental health system and other agencies, State education and health departments, which have the most frequent contact with children, were almost always excluded from coordination programs. The Federal Child and Adolescent Service System Program, described in chapter 10 of this background paper, was established in 1984 to help State mental health agencies coordinate care for one segment of the population of children with mental health problems—those who are severely emotionally disturbed.

CONCLUSION

The educational system, the general health care system, the child welfare system, and the juvenile justice system present important opportunities to identify and help troubled children. Yet evidence suggests that the mental health problems of children involved with these systems are often poorly treated or not treated at all (358,595,645).

The variety of mental health programs potentially available to children would appear to require that such services be integrated across mo-

dalities, providers, settings, and systems although in many cases there may be few services to integrate. The variety of mental health programs also suggests that evaluation of any one intervention program is likely to yield an incomplete picture of the nature and effectiveness of children's mental health care. Variables such as coordination of programs should be taken into account in the assessment of that care.

Part IV: Effectiveness of Services

Chapter 8
Effectiveness of Therapies

Chapter 8
Effectiveness of Therapies

INTRODUCTION

Although the scientific evaluation literature on child treatment is inadequate to answer many policy questions, an increasing amount of research on the effectiveness of children's mental health treatment is available. The fundamental conclusion that professional mental health treatment leads to significantly better outcomes than no treatment across age groups is supported by a substantial research base on the effectiveness of mental health treatment in general (38,484,616,647). Children's mental health treatments cannot be directly equated with treatments for adults (8), but general research tests some of the fundamental assumptions of treatment. Furthermore, there is an extensive theoretical rationale concerning treatment for children's mental disorders (see ch. 5). In many cases, such theory and data are supportive of child treatment interventions, even in the absence of applied research.

To assess current scientific understanding of what is known about the effectiveness of mental health intervention for children, this chapter first discusses reviews of the research that consider the effectiveness of psychotherapies for children in general. Available reviews of psychotherapy outcome research differ in the range of therapies they include within their purview—some including studies of family therapies, for example, and

others not; some including studies of group therapy and others limited to studies of individual therapy. By including studies of a variety of modalities, these reviews analyze the question of whether therapy in general can be effective with troubled children. This question is important because, currently, it is therapy in general that is reimbursed, not particular therapies.

The second part of this chapter examines research on the effectiveness of specific therapies described in chapter 5: behavioral therapy, cognitive therapy, group therapy, family therapy, crisis intervention, and psychopharmacological (drug) therapy.

It should probably be noted that for the most part the scientific literature contains evaluations of the effectiveness of therapies for mental *disorders* (see ch. 3) rather than subclinical mental health problems (see ch. 4); consequently, it is the effectiveness of therapies for diagnosable disorders which is reviewed in this chapter. Some services for subclinical mental health problems come under the rubric of prevention and mental health interventions in non-mental-health settings such as schools, homes, and the juvenile justice system; the effectiveness of such services is reviewed in chapter 9.

EFFECTIVENESS OF CHILD PSYCHOTHERAPY IN GENERAL AND METHODOLOGICAL ISSUES

Nearly 30 years separate the first review of child psychotherapy outcome research (382) from the most recent (104). Not surprisingly, the latest reviews of child psychotherapy outcome research in general have shown greater methodological sophistication, incorporating the more rigorous meta-analytic techniques (387,552,616) to paral-

lel an improved methodological soundness in the studies reviewed. Later reviews also indicate that, in general, treatment for children's mental health problems is more effective than no treatment. However, methodological problems persist, and the conclusions of the reviews should be viewed somewhat cautiously.

Reviews of Child Psychotherapy Outcome Research

Levitt (1957, 1963)

The first major efforts to assess children's mental health treatment were Levitt's (382,383) reviews of child psychotherapy outcome research. Levitt aggregated across available studies the percentages of children who were judged to have improved following treatment. Since most of these studies did not include control groups, he compared the aggregate percentage of treated children who improved to the aggregate percentage of untreated children who improved (derived from two studies).

In his 1957 review (382), Levitt concluded that an estimated 67 percent of treated children had improved at the close of treatment and that 78 percent of treated children had improved at followup; Levitt also found, however, that 72.5 percent of untreated children had improved. These observations suggested that, in general, child psychotherapy for mental health problems did not have an advantage over no treatment. Levitt's 1963 update (383) yielded similar results. Levitt wrote:

> . . . the inescapable conclusion is that available evaluation studies do not furnish a reasonable basis for the hypothesis that psychotherapy facilitates recovery from emotional illness in children.

Levitt's conclusion can be criticized on several grounds. Levitt's estimate of the improvement in untreated children might not have been valid. Levitt derived the estimate of "improvement without treatment" from two studies with questionable methodology (43); and these studies might not have been comparable on several grounds to other treatment outcome studies (280). Furthermore, most of the untreated children were children who received a diagnostic assessment but did not continue with psychotherapy. There might have been systematic differences, aside from treatment, between these children and the treated children. The children who did not receive psychotherapy after diagnosis might have had a greater ability to cope, found other help for their problems, or found the diagnostic contact sufficient treatment (43,106,280). It is also possible that the children in the untreated control groups received mental health treatment somewhere other than at the study site.

Even if Levitt's analytic methods were not suspect, the studies he reviewed might not be representative of the current state of child psychotherapy. The studies he reviewed were done in the 1930s, 1940s, and 1950s. Therapy techniques in those years differed in many ways from later techniques, and the populations studied might have been different from current clinical populations (43). Furthermore, the methods used in psychotherapy outcome studies in those years were primitive in comparison to contemporary methods.

Tramontana (1980)

In a review of the literature on the effectiveness of psychotherapy for adolescents, Tramontana (637) derived estimates of percentage improved similar to Levitt's. Overall, including both individual and group therapy, Tramontana found a median positive outcome rate of 75 percent with psychotherapy and 39 percent without psychotherapy. He questioned the meaningfulness of these figures, however, since the outcomes were so variable across studies—reflecting the variety of factors that influence adolescent therapy outcome. Most of the studies Tramontana reviewed looked at group therapy. Two of them are discussed further below in conjunction with a discussion of group therapy for adolescents.

Smith, Glass, and Miller (1980)

Smith, Glass, and Miller (616) examined 500 controlled studies in their 1980 meta-analysis of psychotherapy. This review was distinguished by its inclusion of controlled studies only and by its taking into account differences in the strength of the treatment effect (effect size) across studies. Critics of the review claim that it lumps together too many different kinds of studies and includes studies of poor as well as good design (174). In fact, Smith and his colleagues attempted to control for this problem by classifying studies according to methodological criteria (647). Although most of the studies examined treatment of adults, approximately 50 of the studies assessed treatment of children or adolescents.

The Smith, et al., 1980 meta-analysis found significantly better outcomes for patients who were treated with psychotherapy than for controls. The investigators concluded that the average person who receives therapy is better off at the end of it than 80 percent of the persons who do not.

Smith, et al., did not analyze the effectiveness of child psychotherapy separately from adult psychotherapy. In a correlational analysis, however, they found that patients' age had little effect on treatment outcome. This finding must be viewed cautiously. The treatment effects of the approximately 50 child and adolescent studies were not analyzed separately from the original 500 studies, and these 50 studies represent a subsample much smaller than the larger group.

Casey and Berman (1985)

Casey and Berman (104) reviewed 75 studies of child psychotherapy outcome dating from 1952 to 1983. They restricted their sample to studies that used a control group of untreated children from the same general population as the treated children. The sample excluded studies examining treatment of adolescents. Behavioral therapy was used in 56 percent of the studies Casey and Berman examined, cognitive-behavioral therapy in 21 percent, and nonbehavioral therapy (psychodynamic, client-centered, mixed, and unclassifiable) in 48 percent. (Some of the studies examined more than one form of treatment, so these figures add to more than 100 percent.)

Using meta-analytic techniques similar to those used by Smith, et al. (616), Casey and Berman (104) found that, overall, the average child receiving psychotherapy was better off after treatment than two-thirds of control children. This treatment effect is comparable to the treatment effect found by Smith, et al. (616), and others reviewing adult psychotherapy. Casey and Berman found little evidence either that one modality of treatment differed from any other in overall effectiveness, or that individual treatment differed from group treatment. Surprisingly, outcomes for children whose parents were treated concurrently did not differ from those of children whose parents were not treated. In general, treatment had a larger effect on problems related to fear and anxiety than on problems involving self-esteem, social adjustment, or global adjustment. The research was insufficient to allow any conclusions matching specific treatment modalities to specific problems or diagnoses.

In general, Casey and Berman concluded that ". . . clinicians and researchers need not be hesitant about defending the merits of psychotherapy for children" (104). The conclusions of Casey and Berman must be reviewed somewhat cautiously however, since only 24 percent of the 75 studies they reviewed clearly used children who were seeking treatment as subjects; most of the rest used "school children not seeking treatment" or "community volunteers for special projects" who were in mental distress but who had not sought treatment. Thus, it is not clear how representative of actual treatment situations their results are.

Methodological Issues

Clinicians and researchers have expressed two major concerns about analyses that aggregate results across different types of treatment as the reviews discussed above have done. One concern is that the research base has too many deficiencies to allow generalizations about the effectiveness of child psychotherapy. Several discussions of the effectiveness of child psychotherapy from Levitt (382) to Kazdin (336) detail the lack of methodologically sound research on the efficacy of child psychotherapy. Among the deficiencies mentioned are the absence or inadequacy of control groups; inadequate or misguided measurement of therapeutic, intervening, and outcome variables; lack of specific description of subjects, treatment, and outcome; heterogeneity of subjects; and failure to assess the effect of psychotherapy independently of other interventions (8,43, 275,280,336,637).

The other major concern is that an overall estimate of the effectiveness of child psychotherapy may have little relevance for clinical practice and mental health policy, because so much seems to depend on a number of mediating factors that influence both children's problems and treatments (see, e.g., 43,280,561,637). Thus, Levitt's (382) review found that the percentage of child patients who improved at close of treatment ranged from 43 to 86 percent across studies, while Tramontana's (637) review found that the percentage improved ranged from 35 to 100 percent. In Casey and Berman's (104) review, the standard deviation exceeded mean effect size, an indication of great variability.

The paucity of good research reflects in part the difficulties of introducing methodological rigor to the study of child psychotherapy (8). Many design features of treatment studies that would be desirable on methodological grounds (e.g., random assignment to treatment or control groups) are rejected as infeasible logistically or questionable ethically (647,719), although there is disagreement about the true extent of logistical and ethical problems. Another obstacle to mental health research in general is the difficulty of specifying what the treatment is, since psychotherapy is often tailored to the specific theoretical orientation of the therapist, the personalities of the therapist and patient, the conditions under which therapy takes place, and, for children's therapy, the developmental stage of the child.

Summary

In summary, research reviews which aggregate a variety of treatments and problems yield mixed evidence for the effectiveness of child psychotherapy. Levitt (382,383) found little difference between treated and nontreated children, but there are serious reservations about the analytic method he used and the studies he reviewed. Smith, et al. (616), found a positive effect of psychotherapy over all ages, with no significant correlation of age with treatment effect; however, they did not analyze studies of child and adolescent treatment separately from studies of adult treatment. Casey and Berman (104) found that treated children had outcomes better than two-thirds of untreated children, but their conclusions must be tempered by the fact that the majority of studies they reviewed did not use actual patients.

EFFECTIVENESS OF SPECIFIC THERAPIES

A refrain resembling the one familiar in adult psychotherapy research seems even more apt for research in child psychotherapy (8,43,280). The important question may not be about the effectiveness of child psychotherapy in general but about:

1. what specific psychotherapy is effective;
2. under what conditions;
3. for which children;
4. at which developmental level;
5. with which problems;
6. under what environmental conditions; and
7. with which concomitant parental, family, environmental, or systems interventions?

The following sections discuss reviews of the research on the effectiveness of specific psychotherapies identified in chapter 5: behavioral therapy, cognitive therapy, group therapy, family therapy, crisis intervention, and psychopharmacological (drug) therapy. Although considerable research has been done for some treatments, such as several types of behavior therapy and some specific pharmacological agents, no research reviews focus specifically on psychodynamic therapy; therefore, a discussion of the effectiveness of psychodynamic therapy is not included.

Effectiveness of Individual Therapy

Behavioral Therapy

Perhaps because of the specificity of behavioral therapy, there are few assessments of the overall effectiveness of behavioral therapy with children. Most studies have investigated the effectiveness of a given behavioral technique for a given problem with a given population in a given context. An exception is Casey and Berman's (104) calculation of an overall treatment effect size across 37 studies of behavioral therapy. Casey and Berman found that behaviorally treated children had better outcomes than 96 percent of untreated children, although treated children had better outcomes than only 55 percent of untreated children when outcome measures that closely resembled the activities of therapy itself (e.g., the number of positive behaviors) were omitted. Behavioral therapy was also one of the modalities represented in the Smith, et al. (616), review.

The effectiveness of specific behavioral treatments for specific problems identified in chapter 3 is briefly reviewed below.

Developmental Disorders.—For children with pervasive developmental disorder (PDD), behavioral treatments have been developed both to increase appropriate behaviors and to decrease maladaptive behaviors (554). Reviews of the research have supported the effectiveness of operant conditioning for teaching PDD children appropriate behaviors such as language and self-care and academic skills although progress is typically slow (252). One difficulty with behavioral treatments is that they often do not generalize beyond the site of treatment. A child learning a skill in a day treatment program may not maintain the learning at home. Although methods of addressing this problem are being developed, further work is needed.

Behavior Disorders.—Some studies of behavioral approaches to the treatment of attention deficit disorder with hyperactivity (ADD-H) suggest that behavioral approaches have had real success in reducing off-task behavior, overactivity, and other problem behaviors and in increasing attention and academic performance (14,29,473). Yet

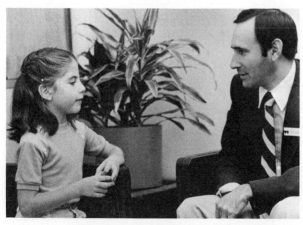

Photo credit: Charter Colonial Institute, Newport News, VA

A variety of treatment modalities, including individual therapy, are used to treat children's mental health problems.

other evidence raises concerns about whether behavioral therapy's effectiveness for ADD-H generalizes to settings beyond the treatment setting, about the duration of the treatment effect (556), and about the possible distracting effect of the rewards used in behavior modification (81). Furthermore, Abikoff and Gittleman (4) found that behavioral treatment of children with ADD-H only reduced aggressiveness; it did not reduce attention deficits, hyperactivity, or impulsivity (555). Abikoff and Gittleman's study suggests that further evaluation is needed to understand the clinical usefulness of behavioral treatment of hyperactivity.

The overall effectiveness of behavior modification for children with conduct disorders is difficult to assess because of the great variation in conduct-disordered behaviors (e.g., from truancy to assault), the great effect that a child's developmental level has on the types of conduct-disordered behaviors exhibited, and the great variation in the severity of conduct disorders. Studies of treatment for younger, less severely disordered children tends to focus on classroom interventions and parent training programs. A number of studies have shown that reinforcement techniques based in the classroom and/or at home have reduced disruptive behavior at school (27).

Parent training programs to reduce conduct-disordered behavior have helped reduce a child's disruptive, difficult behaviors in many families (468). In one effective parent training program (497), parents learned behavioral strategies in a parent training group and made behavioral assessments and changes in their parenting behavior at home. An average of 60-percent reduction in the target disruptive behaviors was achieved.

Emotional Disorders.—Research on behavioral treatment of emotional disorders has been largely restricted to laboratory treatment of specific phobias, a subset of anxiety disorders. One recent review of the outcome research (252) found ample evidence for the effectiveness of modeling procedures but not for reciprocal inhibition or operant conditioning, for treating phobias. The effectiveness of modeling procedures with children diagnosed with other anxiety disorders has not been demonstrated; nor has it been shown that treatment has a lasting effect in a child's normal environment. Behavioral treatment of anxiety disorders is promising, but further research is needed before conclusions about its effectiveness can be made with certainty.

Psychophysiological Disorders.—Evidence for the effectiveness of behavioral treatments for psychophysiological disorders tends to be greater when there is a behavioral component to the disorder. Evidence for the effectiveness of behavioral treatment of Tourette's syndrome (598) and other stereotyped movement disorders is limited.

Evidence for the effectiveness of various behavioral treatments for enuresis (lack of control over urination) is more encouraging. A number of studies have been conducted with several of the behavioral treatments (147). Mowrer's (450) bell-and-pad treatment achieved complete success in 75 percent of studied cases, although 41 percent relapsed when examined at followup (147). Of individuals who relapsed and were retreated, 68 percent achieved lasting success. Strengthening the reinforcement, self-control, or practice components of the bell-and-pad treatment have been found to increase the success rate (147). Most studies examining operant conditioning methods for treating enuresis have found evidence for the success of this method as well (252).

With encopresis (lack of control over defecation), operant conditioning has been successful in several studies, although the total number of children studied has been small (147).

Some evidence exists for the effectiveness of operant conditioning to promote weight gain in patients with anorexia nervosa, but research on behavioral treatment mostly fails to consider the help these patients need with psychological and social aspects of the disorder (54). Behavioral treatment of bulimia has been studied too little for an overall assessment to be made.

Cognitive Therapy

During the past 15 years, the amount of research evaluating cognitive therapies for children often combined with behavioral approaches has increased dramatically (301,341). Cognitive models of treatment have been developed for problems including hyperactivity and conduct disorder, which have often been considered resistant to other treatments. Cognitive therapy and related methods are important approaches in child treatment, because they are closely tied to theory and research in developmental psychology; therefore, they deserve careful assessment (336,399,510,674).

Kendall and Braswell's (341) volume on cognitive-behavioral therapy comprehensively reviews much of the research on this method. The review treats separately two different forms of cognitive-behavioral therapy: self-instructional training and problem-solving. After reviewing nearly 30 studies, Kendall and Braswell concluded that self-instructional training has been shown to be successful with several types of mental health problems. Studies have shown a positive effect of treatment on children's fears, hyperactivity, disruptive behavior, and general self-control. Outcomes were most successful when self-instructional training was combined with operant conditioning, a form of behavioral therapy.

Kendall and Braswell found that much less research has been conducted on problem-solving cognitive approaches, yet much of the research that has been conducted finds successful outcomes such as decreases in disruptive behavior and increases in prosocial behavior.

Cognitive-behavioral therapies were also included in Casey and Berman's (104) review of child psychotherapy outcome studies. Fourteen studies of cognitive-behavioral therapies showed on average that treated children fared better than 81 percent of untreated children, although this figure may be invalid because of the inclusion of outcome measures resembling the therapy (e.g., cognitive functioning rather than behavior).

The conclusion that cognitive and related therapies have been shown to be effective must be qualified in several ways. First, there are some questions about the clinical relevance of some studies, since many of the children have been selected rather than randomly assigned, and many of the outcomes have been measured by scores on tests of cognitive functioning rather than by changes in actual problem behavior (301,336,341). Several studies, however, do show positive effects with clinical populations (336,341). Second, successful outcomes do not always generalize beyond the training situation to the classroom or home, although studies that have included operant conditioning methods or that have broadened the scope of the treatment have often achieved better generalization effects (81,341). Third, aggressive behavior has been especially resistant to cognitive methods (341).

Recent research has investigated such variables as age, developmental level, and cognitive styles of children to help explain differences in outcome and to help tailor cognitive therapies to the requirements of different children (81,341). In a similar vein, Kazdin (336) has noted that studies of more intensive courses of cognitive therapy, with greater focus on specific clinical problems, are needed to test their clinical potential completely.

Effectiveness of Group Therapy

As noted in chapter 5, group therapy for adolescents differs from group treatment for younger children. Child group therapy tends to rely on group play and activities, while adolescent group therapy is more of a "talking" therapy. The literature on each has been discussed in separate reviews. Group therapy has also been included in reviews by Smith, et al. (616), and Casey and Berman (104).

Group Therapy With Prepubescent Children

Abramowitz (5) has reviewed the outcome research on group therapy with prepubescent children. The literature reviewed included studies using verbal approaches (39 percent), play and activity approaches (37 percent), and behavior modification (24 percent). The studies focused on treatment of immature or problem behavior, social isolation or withdrawal, poor self-concept, or academic underachievement. Outcome measures focused chiefly on improvement in personality variables, appropriateness of behavior, interpersonal relations, and academic performance. Abramowitz found that about one-third of the studies demonstrated positive effects of group therapy, one-third had a mixture of positive, negative, and null results, and one-third found no effects of treatment. The generalizability of this evidence must be questioned, however, since most of the outcome studies in Abramowitz's review investigated group therapy that lasted only 10 to 15 sessions and so may not apply to therapy

which lasts longer. Many clinicians argue that a number of initial sessions are needed for a group to "jell" and develop sufficient intimacy for effective therapeutic work to be done (722).

Casey and Berman's (104) review of child psychotherapy included a separate treatment effect size for 33 studies of group treatment. Casey and Berman found that the average child treated in group therapy had a better outcome than 50 percent of untreated children. However, their review does not provide information on the nature of the group treatment; thus, it is difficult to determine if the 33 studies reviewed by Casey and Berman are any more representative than those reviewed by Abramowitz. A fair conclusion is that the full range of child group therapy has not yet been adequately assessed.

Group Therapy With Adolescents

As noted earlier in this chapter, most of the treatment outcome studies in Tramontana's (637) review of adolescent therapy utilized group therapy. Although most of the studies in the Tramontana review were methodologically flawed, two of the studies that evaluated the effectiveness of adolescent group therapy were relatively rigorous. In a study by Persons (503), institutionalized delinquents of both sexes receiving a combination of individual and group psychotherapy were compared with adolescents receiving the standard institutional regimen. The group therapy combined directive and nondirective elements. Persons found positive effects of treatment on anxiety, other psychopathology, academic performance, and antisocial behavior within the institution and at followup in the community. Treated youths also showed better outcomes on measures of employment and recidivism. In a study of a similar population, Redfering (529,530) contrasted institutionalized delinquent adolescents (girls only) receiving short-term group counseling to a nontreated group. At the end of 11 weeks of treatment, the girls in therapy had greater positive changes in self-concept and feelings about parents and peers. Over time, significant differences in parental and self ratings were maintained. Also, treated girls were released more frequently from the institution and recommitted less frequently.

Effectiveness of Family Therapy

Family therapy to deal with children's mental health problems has gained increasing use by clinicians. Family systems theory was found to be useful by more than 60 percent of child therapists in a survey by Koocher and Pedulla (365). Yet outcome studies of family therapy have rarely been included in generic reviews of treatment such as those by Smith, et al. (616), and Casey and Berman (104). Their lack of inclusion speaks both to the newness of family therapy and its status as a conceptually different form of treatment.

Gurman and Kniskern's Overview (1978)

In the most comprehensive review of the family therapy outcome literature, Gurman and Kniskern (267) identified over 200 outcome studies on marital and family therapy. Most of the studies reviewed by Gurman and Kniskern (267) did not identify a child as the patient and will not be considered here (although therapy with parents alone can be helpful to children). Of the studies in which a child was identified as the patient, Gurman and Kniskern (267) reviewed studies of behaviorally based family treatment separately from studies of nonbehavioral family therapies. They also treated studies which used "no treatment" control groups separately from those studies which did not compare families receiving family therapy to families receiving no treatment. Gurman and Kniskern (267) judged that most of the controlled studies they reviewed were well designed.

In the only five studies of behavioral family therapy with children as identified patients, and which used control groups, those children and/or families who received treatment had more positive outcomes than those who received no treatment. Behavioral family therapy led to improvement in the parents' and observers' ratings of children in the majority of uncontrolled studies as well.

In 60 percent of controlled studies of nonbehavioral family therapy, treatment led to more favorable outcomes than no treatment. Because these studies did not include long-term followup, however, the effects of treatment over a longer period of time are not known. Finally, in 19 uncontrolled studies of nonbehavioral family therapy in which children or adolescents were iden-

tified as the patients, 71 percent of treated children and/or families improved, while 29 percent either did not improve or deteriorated. In summary, most studies reviewed in Gurman and Kniskern's comprehensive evaluation found that, in general, family therapy was better than no treatment. Questions remain, however, about the representativeness of the treatments and samples in the studies that Gurman and Kniskern reviewed (267). In addition, their reviews did not speak to the efficacy of family therapy for specific childhood mental health problems.

Effectiveness of Family Therapy With Conduct-Disordered and Delinquent Children

Some researchers have focused on the effectiveness of family therapy with specific childhood mental health problems (268). Two prominent research groups have investigated family therapy for conduct-disordered and delinquent children and adolescents (268,336).

Behavioral family treatments of conduct-disordered children have been extensively investigated by Patterson and associates with over 200 families in studies spanning two decades. Patterson's family intervention, a form of parent training based on social learning principles, has been found to be effective in reducing aggressive and antisocial behavior both in the home (488,493, 495,681,710) and in the classroom (496). Positive effects have also been found in the behavior of siblings and in the mental health of mothers of the identified patients (493,494).

The Functional Family Therapy program of Parsons and Alexander—a cognitive-behavioral family treatment of delinquent adolescents—led not only to an improvement in family interaction (485), but also to a decrease in recidivism (16). Improved family interaction was correlated with declining recidivism. A followup 2½ to 3 years later revealed that siblings of the original identified patients had a reduced number of court contacts as well (356).

While family treatments of conduct-disordered children and youths appear promising, questions remain about the effectiveness of these models of treatment across the broad range of children with conduct disorders. More severely disadvantaged, troubled families have been found to benefit much less than other families from parent management training (336). Similarly, one criticism of Parsons and Alexander's work is that many of the families treated were of the Mormon faith, which stresses family and community cohesiveness and may have provided an unusual impetus for coping with problem behavior (268).

Effectiveness of Family Therapy With Children With Psychophysiological Disorders

Minuchin and colleagues (442,443,444) have studied the effectiveness of family therapy for children with psychophysiological disorders such as anorexia nervosa and chronic illnesses such as diabetes and asthma. They found improvement both in measures of psychosocial functioning and in measures specific to the patients' physical problems (e.g., weight in patients with anorexia nervosa, respiratory functioning in asthmatics). In one study, Schwartz, et al. (268), found improved psychosocial functioning and control of eating in bulimic children treated with family therapy. The lack of control groups in studies of family therapy for children's psychophysiological disorders necessitates caution in interpreting the results, but the achievement of therapeutic results on several fronts with patients often considered unlikely to improve without treatment suggests the potential effectiveness of family therapy.

Summary: Effectiveness of Family Therapy

In general, family therapy outcome studies provide preliminary evidence for the effectiveness of family therapy with many children and families, despite a number of methodological limitations. Studies with some specific populations, such as conduct-disordered children and adolescents, show particular promise. Further research would be necessary to determine when family therapy is most appropriate and to allow knowledgeable matching between type of child, type of disorder, and specific family therapy models and techniques.

Effectiveness of Crisis Intervention

Few studies have evaluated the outcome of crisis intervention. Those studies that have been identified as evaluations have generally focused on adult populations and have not isolated the effectiveness of crisis intervention for child patients. Furthermore, methodological shortcomings limit the conclusions that can be drawn from these studies. Homebuilders, the program discussed in chapter 5 as exemplifying crisis intervention, was evaluated only in terms of its cost-effectiveness and success in avoiding outside placement of patients (350), not in terms of patient functioning. Outside placement was avoided for 90 percent of patients with an estimated cost savings of over $3,200 per patient.

Effectiveness of Psychopharmacological (Drug) Therapy

The effectiveness of psychopharmacological agents in treating childhood disorders can only meaningfully be assessed separately for each pharmacological treatment. The various classes of drug treatment have such contrasting purposes and therapeutic effects that it is impossible to discuss them as a whole. In assessing these medications, the evidence for each intended therapeutic effect must be considered and weighed against the medications' side effects.

Stimulants

The use of stimulant drugs to treat ADD and ADD-H is by far the most common application of psychopharmacological therapy in children, and its effectiveness with children has been researched more than any other drug treatment. Researchers have differentiated the effects of stimulants on specific cognitive functions, academic achievement, social behavior, personality variables, and mood (96). Most research has been focused on short-term effects, but medium and long-term effects of stimulants have also received attention.

Cantwell and Carlson (96) found 15 laboratory experiments demonstrating that several different stimulants successfully aided children with ADD-H in tests of attention, impulsivity, distractibility, motor restlessness, short-term memory, and new learning. These results, however, are not necessarily relevant outside the laboratory.

The effects of stimulants on academic achievement by hyperactive children has been assessed by a number of studies. Barkley and Cunningham (42) reviewed 120 studies of the effect of stimulant drugs on academic achievement, although only 17 of the studies used objective academic measures. Few positive effects of stimulants on academic achievement were found, and those that were found may have reflected the influence of the drugs on school examinations and not on daily learning. Followup studies supported these findings. Thus, there is some evidence for the effectiveness of stimulants on attention deficits, but little evidence that the use of stimulants to treat ADD-H is associated with academic improvement.

Teachers and parents have noted improvements in social behavior in children treated with stimulants for hyperactive and disruptive behavior, (121). Recent research has found parallel effects on some symptoms of ADD-H in adolescents (673), yet methodological difficulties and the developmental differences between adolescents and children prevent any firm conclusions about the effectiveness of stimulants at this time with adolescents with ADD-H.

Although stimulant drugs achieve good short-term results in children with ADD-H, the limited research findings regarding long-term results are much less impressive (526). Available studies have compared children who have been treated continuously for a number of months with children who have had less or no drug treatment, and they show few long-term positive effects of stimulants (526). Some studies suggest that adolescents who have received stimulant treatment sometime during childhood have fewer symptoms of ADD-H than those who have not received stimulant treatment, but that they are still prone to antisocial behavior, poor peer relationships, low self-esteem, and academic problems (279).

Concerns about the side effects of stimulant treatment focus on: 1) possible retardation of physical growth (568), 2) negative effects on learning (628), 3) drug dependence or later drug abuse, and 4) euphoriant effects. A panel appointed by the Food and Drug Administration evaluated the available evidence and concluded that stimulants may have a minor suppressive effect on growth when prescribed in the average-to-high range of dosage. Rapoport (526) addressed the concern about the effects of stimulants on learning and

concluded, after reviewing six studies, that stimulant drugs seem neither to enhance nor retard learning significantly in children with ADD-H. The connection to drug dependence and later drug abuse and the euphoriant effects of stimulants on children have been determined not to be problems (121,658), although some believe that these issues have not been settled conclusively (121).

Neuroleptics

As noted in chapter 5, neuroleptic medication—sometimes called antipsychotic medication—is used not as a treatment to reverse a disorder, but rather as a means of reducing troublesome symptoms associated with a disorder. Neuroleptic medication is prescribed most frequently to control aggressive, assaultive, hyperactive, socially inappropriate, and difficult to manage behavior in severely impaired children, including children with PDD and especially children with mental retardation (390).

The effects of neuroleptic medications with severely disturbed children have been evaluated in a number of studies (714). Most studies have found positive effects of neuroleptics on many outcome measures of behavior, but as Winsberg and Yepes (714) state, these outcomes suggest that neuroleptics ". . . appear useful only in the management of psychotic children, making them less withdrawn, less overactive, less anxious, less agitated and more tractable . . . ." Two studies by Campbell and associates (90,91) also found positive effects of neuroleptics for severely disturbed children in a behavioral (operant) learning paradigm, probably because of their effect of reducing inappropriate responses (92).

One neuroleptic, haloperidol (Haldol®), has been shown to be effective in reducing the tics and other symptoms of Tourette's syndrome, although there are few controlled studies (598). Neuroleptics have also been used in low doses to treat ADD-H; however, in comparative studies, stimulants have usually outperformed neuroleptics for treatment of hyperactivity and are generally preferred clinically (714).

A number of side effects of neuroleptics have been documented and are of concern. The sedative effect of neuroleptics appears to impair cognitive functioning in children who are already cognitively impaired (17,75). Evidence for this effect, however, has been limited to nonclinical populations. Other short-term side effects can include drowsiness; blurred vision; and moderate motor dysfunction like tremors, occasional mood changes, and changes in urinary behavior. The long-term side effects of most concern are medication-induced movement disorders, especially those that emerge when the medication is stopped (220), and, in a few cases, tardive dyskinesia (498).

The proportion of children treated with neuroleptics who develop side effects is unknown; in the few studies available, estimates of the prevalence of the different side effects of neuroleptics vary widely. Conners and Werry (121) note that most side effects are not serious, and those that are (e.g., tardive dyskinesia) are infrequent and occur only with high doses or prolonged use. It appears, however, that the decision to use neuroleptics with severely disordered children must be made judiciously and the dosage must be carefully controlled. Some side effects—especially the general "quasi-sedative" effect (714)—have provoked concern among many professionals and parents about the frequent use of drugs (622).

Antidepressants

Well-conducted research on the effectiveness of antidepressant treatment of childhood depression has increased in the past several years, but definitive information awaits the completion of more studies. In a recent review, Puig-Antich and colleagues (518) note that none of the more rigorous studies so far have shown antidepressants to be better than placebos across samples of depressed children, although certain subgroups of depressed children have responded to antidepressants. Such issues as appropriate dosage, effect of a child's developmental level, and clinical improvements due apparently to placebo effects complicate conclusions about the effectiveness of antidepressants in treating childhood depression.

In addition to being used to treat depression, antidepressants have been used to treat enuresis, ADD-H, separation anxiety, and school phobia. The antienuretic effect of antidepressants may be entirely separate from their antidepressant action, but numerous studies have found antidepressants to be effective in reducing, though not curing, enuresis (527). Antidepressants are somewhat effective in treating ADD-H, but generally less effective than stimulants (528). Antidepressants have been used successfully in combination with psychosocial (behavioral, cognitive, and psychodynamic) treatments to treat school phobia (233), and separation anxiety caused, according to the investigator's theory, by biochemical disturbances not associated with depression (232).

Although the side effects of antidepressants can be dangerous in some children (121), the immediate side effects (e.g., dry mouth, drowsiness, sweating) of moderate to low doses of antidepressants mainly cause discomfort (527). In higher dosages, antidepressant medication can have cardiovascular side effects, but these can be minimized by adhering to strict limits on dosage level (518). Use of antidepressants with suicidally depressed children is risky, because overdoses of these drugs are extremely toxic (527). Conners and Werry (121) state:

> . . . of all the psychotropic drugs commonly used in children, the tricyclics call for the greatest caution.

CONCLUSION

Although methodological problems plague research on the effectiveness of children's mental health treatments, considerable evidence has accumulated to suggest the effectiveness of a wide range of modalities of treatment. The most recent review of the effectiveness of child psychotherapy in general (104) found that the average child receiving therapy was better off after treatment than two-thirds of control children, and the authors recommend that professionals not hesitate in defending child psychotherapy's merits. Even this review is limited, however, by the fact that most studies reviewed did not use actual patients in treatment. Many treatments, used widely for a variety of mental health problems, have not yet been evaluated systematically.

With respect to specific treatments, even though an overall assessment of their effectiveness cannot yet be made, several psychosocial therapies have shown promise in a number of studies, especially in some specific problem areas. Thus, for example, behavioral treatment is clearly effective for phobias and enuresis, and cognitive-behavioral therapy is effective for a range of disorders involving self-control (except aggressive behavior). Group therapy has been found to be effective with delinquent adolescents, and family therapy appears to be effective for children with conduct disorders and psychophysiological disorders. Psychopharmacological treatment, while not curative, has been found to have limited effectiveness with children with ADD-H, depression, or enuresis, and also in managing the behavior of children who are severely disturbed. Further, more rigorous research may demonstrate the usefulness of several other treatments for which there is preliminary evidence of effectiveness.

Effectiveness of Treatment and Prevention in Mental Health and Other Settings, and Evaluating the Integration of Mental Health and Other Services

Effectiveness of Treatment and Prevention in Mental Health and Other Settings, and Evaluating the Integration of Mental Health and Other Services

INTRODUCTION

The effectiveness of various settings for children's mental health treatment is of interest to policymakers and was one of the reasons this background paper was requested. Mental health treatment settings vary considerably in intensiveness, restrictiveness, and cost. Therefore, it is valuable to have systematic information about the effectiveness of alternative settings to justify placement, reimbursement, and public policy decisions. Similarly, evidence about the effectiveness of prevention efforts and the integration of services across mental health and other systems is valuable.

Chapter 6 described the mental health settings in which disturbed children receive treatment. Such settings range from inpatient hospital settings to private mental health practices. For those settings that provide a therapeutic milieu or engage mentally disturbed children in treatment for substantial periods of time each week—e.g., hospitals, residential treatment centers (RTCs), and day treatment programs—the setting itself may have an important effect on treatment outcome. Available outcome research on the use of these settings for mental health treatment is reviewed in this chapter.

Chapter 7 described broad-based interventions to identify and treat children's mental health problems within the educational, general health care, child welfare, and juvenile justice systems; it also described efforts to prevent children's mental health problems and to integrate mental health and other services. Because of a lack of research, the effectiveness of treatment in most of the non-mental-health systems cannot be evaluated. Information on outcomes in the child welfare system (e.g., therapeutic foster homes or group homes), for example, is insufficient to be reviewed. There is some research on the effectiveness of interventions in the educational and juvenile justice systems, however, and that research is considered in this chapter. Also reviewed is some of the most rigorous research on prevention programs. There have been very few efforts to evaluate the integration of mental health and other services generally and no such efforts to date for children's mental health services. A planned evaluation of a new Federal effort to integrate services is described in this chapter.

EFFECTIVENESS OF TREATMENT IN SELECTED MENTAL HEALTH TREATMENT SETTINGS

Understanding the respective roles of mental health treatment modalities and treatment settings in therapeutic outcome would be invaluable in designing mental health programs. Unfortunately, the current state of research on outcomes makes it difficult to separate effects due to particular treatment modalities from effects due to the settings in which treatment occurs, or to no treatment. From a methodological perspective, the principal problem is that available research has not used control groups to compare the effectiveness of alternate settings. Disturbed children with similar diagnoses and life circumstances have not been randomly assigned to either a hospital, an RTC, a community mental health center (CMHC), or other outpatient setting giving similar treatments and the children's treatment outcomes subsequently compared.

The effects of some treatment elements such as intensive individual therapy may be easier to disentangle from the settings in which treatment is given, but systematic research that attempts to do this has not been conducted. Consequently, it is difficult to assess the degree to which alternative treatments or alternative settings would have achieved similar or different therapeutic outcomes (580).

Effectiveness of Psychiatric Hospitalization

The most intensive, as well as costly, form of mental health treatment involves inpatient care in a hospital. Although psychiatric hospitals are a type of residential treatment, the services they provide may differ from services provided in nonmedically focused settings such as RTCs. Consequently, a somewhat separate research literature on the effectiveness of psychiatric hospitalization for children has developed (61,245).

Blotcky, et al. (61), reviewed two dozen followup studies of mentally disturbed children under the age of 12 who had been treated in hospital inpatient and other residential psychiatric facilities. One-fifth of the studies were prospective. One-third included adolescents as well as children.

All of the followup studies that Blotcky and colleagues reviewed reported some positive treatment outcomes. The studies concluded, however, that treatment outcomes were primarily associated with the severity of disturbance. That is, they found that over half of the children described as neurotic or exhibiting personality disorders demonstrated long-term positive outcomes following inpatient treatment. More severely impaired children, diagnosed as psychotic (i.e., having disorders involving severely disturbed perceptions

of reality) or neurologically impaired, had somewhat fewer positive outcomes. Outcomes also appeared to be related to variables such as characteristics of the patient other than diagnosis (e.g., intelligence), family factors (parental psychopathology), and, to a lesser extent, treatment variables (e.g., length of stay, aftercare). However, treatment courses were so variable, and periods between discharge and followup so long in most studies reviewed, that inferences about effective elements of inpatient and other residential treatment cannot be made. In many cases, it was impossible to determine whether the treatment setting more resembled a hospital or an RTC.

According to Blotcky, et al., because controlled research has not been done and inpatient followup studies have not compared results of inpatient mental health treatment to either natural course or outpatient treatment, it is difficult to know the relationship between inpatient psychiatric treatment and outcomes.

Gossett, et al. (245), reviewed 22 followup studies of mentally disturbed adolescents who had received inpatient psychiatric treatment, and their conclusions about the effectiveness of such treatment were similar to those of Blotcky, et al. (61). The studies Gossett and colleagues reviewed indicated that the majority of nonpsychotic adolescents who had received inpatient treatment were functioning at an adaptive level several years after discharge. Of psychotic adolescents who had received inpatient treatment, only one-third were adjusted adequately at followup. In general, the less severe and chronic the adolescent patients' initial problems—including level of family psychopathology—the more positive their eventual outcomes, although Gossett, et al.'s review found that aftercare was associated with positive outcomes.

A primary goal of developing this background paper was to respond to questions about the effectiveness and appropriateness of psychiatric hospitalization for children and adolescents. The methodological limitations of available studies of inpatient psychiatric care make firm conclusions difficult. Available studies do not clearly show which components of hospital treatment contribute to successful outcomes. Neither do they allow conclusions about whether children treated as hospital inpatients would have better, worse, or similar outcomes with nonhospital treatment. Because of the methodological limitations of available studies, it is unclear to what extent outcomes for mentally disturbed children treated in hospitals are a function of the children's level of disturbance. In many cases, hospital treatment is a "last resort" for children who have been unsuccessfully treated in other settings. Prospective research controlling for patient characteristics and family variables has not been conducted.

Effectiveness of Residential Treatment Centers

There are many similarities between RTCs and children's psychiatric hospitals, and the findings about effectiveness of RTCs are similar to those for psychiatric hospitals. Several studies have investigated the effects of RTC treatment, chiefly on outcomes measured during or soon after treatment. Unfortunately, however, interpretation of these studies, like studies of inpatient treatment, is limited by the fact that most of the studies lacked control groups.

Whittaker and Pecora (706) reviewed eight studies of RTC treatment. Without exception, the

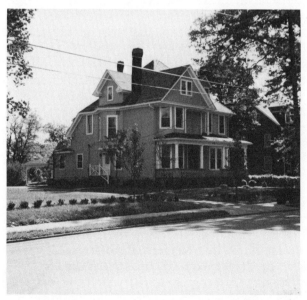

Photo credit: OTA

This group home serves as an intermediate step for adolescent boys who still need supervised care and treatment before returning to their families.

studies found that the majority of children made satisfactory adjustment while still in RTC treatment. Unlike the results for psychiatric hospitals, the evidence for a relationship between severity of a child's problems at admission (or other diagnostic variables) and posttreatment outcome was inconclusive. Following treatment, however, their level of adjustment depended on the quality of the posttreatment environment, the amount of stress or social support (especially family support), quality of parent-child relationships, and family stability. Greater involvement of the family with RTC treatment and with postdischarge planning was also associated with favorable outcomes.

Lewis, et al. (386), performed a followup study of 51 children who had received RTC treatment. Most of these children had been considered improved at the time of discharge, but were rated poorly adjusted at later followup by independent evaluators. The majority of poorly adjusted children had had more than two institutional placements following RTC treatment. Children who had been older at the time of admission to RTC treatment and who had exhibited both psychotic and organic symptoms also tended to have poorer outcomes as did children with disturbed parents, although Lewis, et al., point out that it is impossible to separate possible genetic contributions from environmental contributions to outcome. Lewis and his colleagues note that many of the children in the study completed RTC treatment just prior to adolescence and suggest that poor outcomes for these children might have resulted from the turmoil of adolescence combined with the difficulty of being released into a stressful environment.

Re-ED programs are a type of RTC that appears particularly promising (see ch. 6). In a study by Weinstein (686), data on one Re-ED program, Cumberland House, were gathered from parents, Re-ED teacher-counselors, teachers in the children's regular class, classroom peers, referring agency staff, and from the children themselves. Weinstein's study, considered one of the best of the Re-ED evaluations, found that children who had completed the program had more positive self-concepts, a greater sense of self-control, and better academic performance than a disturbed but untreated control group. The children who had completed the program were rated as improved by Re-ED staff, regular teachers, other professional staff, and parents, but, curiously, not by their peers. Despite their apparent improvement, however, Re-ED children were rated more poorly on most measures than a nontroubled control group.

Other evaluation and followup studies of Re-ED programs have found results such as improved academic achievement, increased prosocial behavior as measured by an antisocial behavior checklist, successful discharge of over 65 percent of residents, improved home and school relationships, and improved school enrollment following treatment, although some school problems continued (606). Since the researchers' assessment measures were sensitive to a wide range of outcomes, many in the community, Weinstein's study provides preliminary support for the Re-ED program model. However, only a few studies have evaluated Re-ED outcomes, so conclusions about the Re-ED program's effectiveness ought to be viewed with caution. Long-term followup data do not yet exist, and measurement of outcome by independent clinicians or other independent observers is lacking.

The outcome research on RTCs, though not extensive or methodologically rigorous, suggests that although most children treated at RTCs improve during treatment, their long-term outcomes may be less positive and depend on the involvement of the family in treatment, the amount of stress in the environment, and the availability of social support. The implication of available research is that the effectiveness of RTC treatment cannot be considered in isolation, but must be evaluated in conjunction with the quality of followup care. Another implication is that coordination between RTCs, community agencies, and the family is necessary. Although Lewis, et al. (386), suggest that the "undoing" of RTC treatment that can happen in the community implies the need for longer RTC treatment, no evidence is available to indicate that longer RTC treatment leads to better outcomes or that longer RTC treatment is superior to RTC treatment combined with adequate followup care.

Effectiveness of Day Treatment

As noted in chapter 6, day treatment is intermediate in intensity between outpatient and 24-hour care, as in psychiatric hospitals or RTCs. As such, it is used both as a less restrictive alternative to inpatient treatment and as a transition from inpatient to outpatient care. Although data on the number of children in day treatment are not available, the number of day treatment centers for children has increased dramatically—concomitantly with the development of CMHCs—from 10 in 1961 to over 350 in 1980 (735). Research on the effectiveness of child day treatment has also increased in recent years, corresponding to the treatment's greater availability, but most of it has not been methodologically rigorous.

Zimet and Farley (735) reviewed six followup studies that evaluated day treatment outcomes for children. The day treatment programs evaluated in the six studies relied on a variety of theoretical orientations (behavioral, psychodynamic, etc.) or combinations of orientations. Zimet and Farley state that the studies they reviewed reported "satisfactory adjustments" in 76 to 90 percent of children receiving day treatment. "Satisfactory adjustments" included outcomes such as improved self-esteem, greater academic achievement, improved social relationships, and more appropriate behavior. Children in day treatment were less likely to be placed in inpatient settings. Younger children generally made greater gains than older children. Results on the effects of parental involvement with children in day treatment were mixed.

Friedman and Quick (208) reported a study in which two groups of children who did not complete a day treatment program (one group completed over 50 days of treatment) were compared to one group of children who did complete the program. Adolescents who had substantial involvement with the multimodality program that was studied had greater academic gains than those with minimal involvement. At followup, 2 years after discharge from treatment, greater involvement with the program appeared to be associated with a lower probability of being a runaway or being institutionalized. According to Friedman and Quick, the group of children who dropped out of day treatment included many chronic runaways and truants "whose behavior was very appropriate while attending, but for whom the program failed to secure consistently good attendance."

Like most treatment outcome research in the field of children's mental health, available studies of day treatment lack methodological rigor. Definitive conclusions about the effectiveness of day treatment, therefore, must await further investigations. Nevertheless, the consistency with which positive outcomes following day treatment have been reported is encouraging.

EFFECTIVENESS OF TREATMENT IN SELECTED NON-MENTAL-HEALTH SYSTEMS

As noted in chapter 7, mental health treatment is sometimes delivered in settings in the educational, health care, child welfare, and juvenile justice systems. A few such interventions that have been evaluated are discussed below. Because of the paucity of evaluation studies of such interventions, the discussion that follows is not comprehensive.

Effectiveness of Treatment in the Educational System

A large investigation of mental health interventions in the school system of Newcastle-upon-Tyne in England was undertaken by Kolvin, et al. (362). Their aim was to compare the effectiveness of a range of different approaches to mental health intervention in a community setting. The investigators identified 574 disturbed children (265 7-year-olds and 309 11-year-olds) in 12 schools and randomly assigned them to a no-treatment control group or to one of four treatment conditions: 1) child group therapy, 2) behavior modification applied to entire classrooms (for older children only), 3) parent guidance, and 4) a nonspecific "nurturance" intervention provided by teacher-aides in school (for younger children only). All the treatments except parent guidance (which took place in the home) were delivered at school. The investigators believed that the school setting allowed them a number of advantages over a clinic setting—a better grasp of the children's social environment, the children's greater familiarity with the setting, and more opportunity for involvement by teachers.

Disturbed children were identified from an index based on a combination of teacher, peer, and self ratings, along with reading scores and attendance records. A control group of nondisturbed children was used for comparison purposes. The experimental and control groups were not entirely comparable, however, because disturbed children had a lower socioeconomic status than nondisturbed children and also had a greater lifetime incidence of broken homes and health problems.

The children in the Newcastle-upon-Tyne study were treated for anywhere from two to five school terms, depending on the intervention condition. Outcome was assessed at the end of treatment, and then at 18 months and 3 years after treatment. All the treatments led to improvement on at least some measures. In general, the group therapy and nurturance approaches led to better results for the younger children, and the behavior modification and group therapy were most effective for the older children. Emotionally disordered children tended to improve more than behavior-disordered children. One important finding was that the effectiveness of the behavioral intervention tended to increase over time, suggesting a "sleeper" effect of treatment. The modality of treatment was a better predictor of success than the sheer duration of treatment.

Effectiveness of Treatment in the Juvenile Justice System

A research program conducted by Massimo and Shore (419,604,605) examined the effect of a "vocationally-oriented psychotherapeutic program" for adolescent delinquent boys. In line with the researchers' understanding of the specific needs of delinquents, this program offered a comprehensive set of interventions that differed greatly from the traditional clinical approach. Job counseling and placement was the first component introduced, and psychotherapeutic contact was added later; the program also included help such as remedial education and aid in managing money.

Outcomes were measured during the 10-month treatment period, and at 2 to 3, 5, and 10 years later. Treated adolescents showed improved adjustment emotionally, academically, and voca-

tionally. Massimo and Shore's work is often cited as a promising multi-intervention program that has shown some success with a difficult-to-treat population.

Studies of behavioral treatment for more severe conduct disorders often take place in juvenile justice settings. Reviews suggest that operant behavioral programs have led to improvement in a number of social, academic, and personal behaviors within the treatment setting (136,170). However, there is little evidence that these behavioral improvements carry over to behavior in natural, community environments (252).

EFFECTIVENESS OF SELECTED PREVENTION EFFORTS

In recent decades, there has been increasing acceptance and support of the concept of services to prevent mental health problems. Preventive mental health efforts have burgeoned and received support on many levels (Federal, State, and community). A solid research base detailing the effectiveness of prevention strategies is just beginning to accumulate. Several fairly rigorous outcome studies have been done, but these studies examine only a minority of the prevention efforts that have been or could be undertaken. To some extent, the paucity of methodologically sound research on the effectiveness of prevention efforts parallels the paucity of rigorous research on the effectiveness of children's mental health services in general. In addition, however, the amount of information currently available about the effectiveness of prevention is limited by difficulties that are specific to prevention outcome research (e.g., the low base rate of certain disorders in the population, the large cost and effort involved in long-term followup studies, and the wide range of target problems and interventions included in the concept of prevention) (281). Nonetheless, available research suggests that certain prevention strategies can be quite effective, both in terms of preventing the development of mental disorders and in promoting mental health and adaptation.

As is noted in chapter 7, prevention programs have taken a number of forms. Such programs have been aimed at almost all of the mental health

problems that fall into the standard diagnostic categories and at the problems associated with environmental risk factors. Moreover, they have occurred in a diverse array of settings (e.g., home, school, mental health centers) and have involved the participation of children and parents, as well as whole families, classrooms, and schools. The wide range of prevention programs which have been implemented and evaluated precludes an exhaustive review of the effectiveness of all types of prevention programs. A selected group of the more rigorous outcome studies is described below.

Effectiveness of Selected Primary Prevention Efforts

As noted in chapter 7, primary prevention efforts are aimed at reducing the incidence of mental health problems in children. Some of these efforts are directed at parents and others at children.

Parent Training Programs

Interventions aimed at reducing the interactional and developmental difficulties often associated with preterm birth and adolescent parenting have been well researched. One research group that used random selection and assignment to treatment and control conditions found that biweekly intervention in the form of home visits designed to facilitate interaction between teenage mothers and their preterm infants improved the

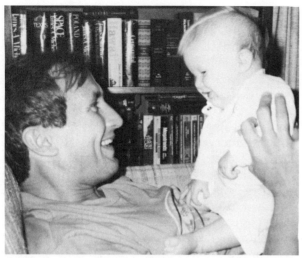

Photo credit: OTA

Studies have shown that programs to encourage healthy parent-child interaction can promote children's mental health.

infants' physical, cognitive, social, and temperamental outcomes (187).

Teen Pregnancy Prevention Programs

Another well-researched prevention effort is "Project Redirection," a large-scale, multisite program aimed at preventing repeat pregnancies and fostering educational and vocational attainment in teenagers. Investigators in one study found significant beneficial effects 1 year after the intervention in terms of lower rates of subsequent pregnancy and higher rates of school enrollment and employment; however, 2 years after the intervention, many of the benefits were no longer apparent (522).

Early Education and Child Development Programs

Among the most widely implemented and extensively researched prevention efforts are the early education intervention programs that originated with Head Start in the mid-1960s. As noted in chapter 7, although these programs were not specifically directed at preventing mental health problems, they have addressed the needs of children at risk for educational and adaptive failures, which have been shown to be associated with later mental health problems (127,514,546,675,699).

The history of evaluation of early education programs is essentially one of initial enthusiasm and excessive optimism, giving way to pessimism and a sense of failure, and ultimately arriving at a more balanced view of what these programs have and have not achieved (731,734). Early pronouncements of the failure of early education programs were, in part, the result of an evaluation known as the "Westinghouse Report," which concluded that Head Start programs produced no lasting gains in cognitive and affective development (113). The Westinghouse Report was widely publicized and generated questions both about the premises of the Head Start program and the validity of outcome measures.

One response to these questions was a general reassessment of the long-term effectiveness of early education programs by the Consortium for Longitudinal Studies (378). This study involved the pooling of original data from 12 investigators who had independently designed and implemented evaluations of early education programs for low-income children in the 1960s. Thus, this study was a joint evaluation of the early education programs' long-term effects. Although all of the early education programs had focused on economically disadvantaged preschool-aged children, they differed in terms of program length, mode of intervention, and program setting (home- or center-based). The evaluations of the programs varied in the extent to which they utilized random assignment to treatment and control conditions.

The study by the Consortium for Longitudinal Studies found that low-income children who had participated in early education programs were significantly more likely than controls to have met school requirements. Participants were less likely to have been assigned to special education classes or to have been retained in a grade. Participants also showed higher IQ and achievement test scores during the first 3 or 4 years following program participation, although differences in IQs of program and control children were not found after this time. Early education was found to have had a lasting effect on attitudes towards achievement —both among the children and their parents. Specifically, program children were found to have a more positive attitude towards achievement and school than controls and their mothers were found to be more satisfied with their children's school performance and to have consistently higher occupational aspirations for them.

In a more recent study of the effects of preschool education through age 19, Berreuter-Clement, et al. (56), found, in addition to the effects on school and attitude found in earlier studies, that by age 19, the preschool group's employment experience was significantly better than the experience of a no-preschool control group.

In general, the studies by the Consortium for Longitudinal Studies and Berreuter-Clement and his colleagues suggest that early education has significant and lasting effects on children's functioning (378). Although the exact mechanisms by which the early education programs lead to positive outcomes are not known, it has been suggested that cognitive, social, and motivational factors were involved. Furthermore, the positive effects of early education programs have been attributed not only to changes produced in the children but, perhaps more importantly, to the effects programs had on parents (6,10,734) and others in the child's environment, including siblings (249) and other social institutions in communities served by the program (77,352,469,671). Such effects illustrate the importance of providing services in the context of children's lives.

The implementation and evaluation of early education intervention projects have important implications for the evaluation of prevention efforts in general. Zigler and Berman (731) emphasize the importance of avoiding the type of overpromising that accompanied Head Start in its early years. Although early intervention has been shown to result in benefits for children and families, it is an error to assume that an early education program alone can eliminate the often pervasive effects of social and economic disadvantage. Furthermore, these authors note, there are problems associated with overstressing change in IQ score as the major criterion of the effectiveness of early education efforts. Although measures of formal cognitive ability are important, benefits in other essential realms of functioning have resulted from these efforts. Zigler and Berman suggest broadly defined "social competence" as a more appropriate measure of outcome (733).

Family Support Programs

Much less is known about the effectiveness of interventions directed at supporting effective functioning in high-risk families than is known about the effectiveness of early education and other programs designed to provide cognitive stimulation to children (594). As evaluations of early education increasingly make clear, however, the most effective interventions are often those that actively involve parents as well as children (77,250). This observation suggests that family support may be a central aspect of promoting children's mental health. Because family support programs are a fairly recent development, few outcome studies of such programs are available. Evaluations of two family support programs described in chapter 7—the Yale Child Welfare Research Program and the Family Support Center Program—are reviewed below.

The Yale Child Welfare Research Program (see ch. 7) is a program aimed at enhancing the functioning of high-risk families. Since its inception, the program has used a matched control group and has undergone several evaluations.

Initial evaluations of the Yale program found that program children (at 30 months of age) showed significantly better language development than the control children; however, control group families were more likely to be self-supporting and to include a father or father-surrogate in their home (516). Five years later, the program families were found to be living in improved socioeconomic circumstances, and program mothers were more likely than control group mothers to be employed and to have fewer total children (539,638). Moreover, at that time, the children in program families were found to have higher IQ scores, better school achievement, and better school attendance than a control sample (638).

The most recent evaluation of the Yale program (594) is a 10-year followup of original program participants and an equivalent control group of parents and children. This evaluation found that 10 years after participating in the Yale program, participating mothers were more likely than control group mothers to be self-supporting, to have achieved higher levels of education, and to have had fewer children. They were also more likely to display self-initiated involvement in their children's schooling. The participating children, although they did not have significantly higher IQ scores than the control group children, had better school attendance, required fewer costly special services, and showed better social and school adjustment. In addition, the program was found to save money; in 1 year, the 15 control group families were found to require approximately $40,000 worth of school services and extrafamilial support services that were not needed by the intervention families.

An evaluation of the Family Support Center Program (FSCP) (see ch. 7) compared FSCP families with a sample of normal families (25). It found that FSCP families had significantly fewer incidents of child abuse, were experiencing less stress, and had developed better parent-child interaction and child care conditions by the end of the program. Greater involvement in the program was correlated with better outcomes. The validity of the findings is limited by the lack of a control group and the fact that half of the FSCP families did not complete all three phases of the program. Also, many of the families participating in FSCP received additional services from other agencies during the course of the intervention.

Effectiveness of Selected Secondary Prevention Efforts

The Primary Mental Health Program (PMHP) is an extensively implemented and evaluated secondary prevention program (126). Although used with children slightly older than the children in Head Start, PMHP is similarly focused on the prevention of educational failure and school maladjustment; PMHP also shares the premise that amelioration of early difficulties has important preventive implications for later mental health problems. Unlike Head Start, PMHP selects for the program children who are already beginning to experience problems.

Since the program's inception, outcome research has been a central component of PMHP. Several studies attest to PMHP's effectiveness in reducing problem behaviors and enhancing competence in high-risk groups (128,694). Attention has also been paid to the long-term effects of participation in PMHP; children have been found to maintain significant gains in adjustment for 1 to 5 years following PMHP intervention (107,394).

In a recent 2- to 5-year followup (107), PMHP children were compared with a "never seen" group (children judged to be well-adjusted at the time of initial screening) and a "least well-adjusted" group (non-PMHP children who were judged by their teachers to be functioning poorly). This study found that the PMHP children maintained, and in some cases solidified further, the gains in adjustment and problem reduction they had made 2 to 5 years earlier. In addition, although PMHP children were often found to be functioning less well than the "never seen" children, they consistently appeared to be better adjusted than the "least well-adjusted" children. This observation suggests that although PMHP did not completely eradicate early detected difficulties, it did significantly prevent the development of serious problems in a high-risk group. Finally, PMHP children were found to perform in the normal range on academic achievement measures at followup, suggesting a sustained and long-term benefit of the intervention.

Summary: Effectiveness of Prevention

Research on the outcomes of prevention programs for specific mental disorders is very undeveloped. There are, however, some fairly rigorous studies on the outcomes of efforts to prevent more broadly defined maladjustment—e.g., PMHP and early education and child development programs. These studies suggest that prevention, or at least reduction, of an incipient mental health problem is a worthwhile and attainable goal.

EVALUATING THE INTEGRATION OF MENTAL HEALTH AND OTHER SERVICES

As difficult as it is, evaluating specific programs is simple compared to evaluating the effects of integrating mental health and other services. In their review of methods for evaluating services integrated across systems, Morrissey, et al. (666), found little solid evidence to support the belief of some investigators (e.g., 262) that organization-level variables predict client-level outcomes. Evaluations of the effects of integrated services on client-level outcomes would require the integration of system, program, and client-level data; studies encompassing all three levels of data are relatively rare in the health and welfare field (666).

At present, there are no reviews of attempts at coordinating mental health and other service systems. The National Institute of Mental Health (NIMH) and grantees of NIMH's Child and Adolescent Service System Program (CASSP) are beginning to develop criteria for evaluating CASSP, a program intended to foster collaboration and integration among mental health and other service systems (see ch. 10). Outcome measures will include States' progress toward a "minimal service set"; the extent to which parents are used as advocates for children; declines in the number of children placed out of State; and other measures of services, leadership, advocacy, and training. However, actual child outcomes will not be part of the evaluation.

CONCLUSION

Methodologically rigorous research comparing the effectiveness of treatment in psychiatric hospitals and other residential settings with similar treatment in outpatient settings is sorely lacking. Despite the limitations of available research, however, certain trends in the data are suggestive—and support particular policy choices. The long-term effectiveness of psychiatric hospitalization and other forms of RTC treatment, for example, appears to be related to the availability of social support mechanisms and mental health services in the posttreatment evironment programs. The effectiveness of mental health treatment in non-mental-health settings may depend on pairing treatment with other interventions like vocational counseling or family support.

Existing models of prevention suggest that effective interventions can be offered through any of several existing systems—including the family, the schools, and health care programs. Not only have many prevention programs led to positive changes in social, emotional, and academic measures, but such programs appear capable of preventing later governmental expenditures through the justice and welfare systems.

What is clear, is that much greater emphasis needs to be placed on evaluations of mental health services offered in a variety of settings, including non-mental-health settings. Assessment of integrated treatment systems could help policymakers decide how to target resources.

Part V: Current Federal Efforts

Chapter 10
Current Federal Efforts

Current Federal Efforts

INTRODUCTION

The complexity of children's mental health problems, the diversity of mental health treatments, and the effectiveness, in general, of treatment have been documented in previous chapters. Despite an incomplete knowledge of the causes of mental health problems in children, it is clear that much can be done to reduce the effects of such problems. Yet substantial data suggest that many children with mental disorders, and at risk of developing such problems, do not have access to adequate treatment services (216,358).

This chapter examines the Federal role in providing mental health services to children. Where possible, it considers that role in the context of the entire mental health system—State, local, and private. The chapter describes specific Federal programs with the greatest relevance to children's mental health services. Such programs relate to financing of children's mental health treatment; coordination of mental health and other services; research and training; and prevention and other services. The chapter concludes that although the roles of State and local governments and the private sector in serving the mental health needs of children could be usefully enhanced, greater Federal involvement may also be desirable.

FEDERAL PROGRAMS THAT SUPPORT MENTAL HEALTH AND RELATED SERVICES FOR CHILDREN

Several Federal programs affect the provision of mental health services to children. The discussion in this chapter emphasizes the programs that have the most direct influence:

- the Alcohol, Drug Abuse, and Mental Health (ADM) block grant program, which provides funds to States for community mental health centers (CMHCs);
- third-party payment programs such as Medicaid, Medicare, and the Civilian Health and Medical Program of the Uniformed Services (CHAMPUS), which are involved, to a greater or lesser degree, in financing children's mental health care;
- related psychological services under the Education for All Handicapped Children Act (Public Law 94-142);
- the Child and Adolescent Service System Program (CASSP) of the National Institute of Mental Health (NIMH), which is intended to coordinate mental health and other services for severely mentally disturbed children; and
- NIMH training, research, and prevention programs.

Federal contributions to these programs in 1985 and, where they can be determined, estimated amounts devoted to children's mental health services in 1985 are shown in table 8. Because funds for children's mental health are commingled with resources for adults and for alcohol, drug abuse, and other health-related programs, the precise amount of Federal resources dedicated to children's mental health is not reliably known. The estimates given, therefore, should be viewed cautiously.

Financing of Mental Health Treatment

When considering the role of the Federal Government in the financing of children's mental health treatment, it is important to note that mental health treatment (for all ages combined) is financed primarily by State Mental Health Agencies (SMHAs). In general, Federal and private sources currently bear less of a burden, although

Table 8.—Federal Contributions to Programs Contributing to Mental Health Services for Children, 1985
(dollars in millions)

Federal program[a]	Total Federal contribution to mental health and other health services	Mental health portion, adults and children	Children's mental health portion	
			Amount	Percent of total mental health portion
Mental health services programs:				
Alcohol, Drug Abuse, and Mental Health (ADM) block grant (1981)	$ 490	$200[b]	NA[c]	NA
10-percent set-aside for new mental health programs for children or other underserved populations (1985)	—	—	$ 10.6 to $20.0[d]	NA
Total.......................................	490	200	NA	NA
NIMH Office of State and Community Liaison...........	13	13	4.7	36%
Child and Adolescent Service System Program (CASSP) (1984)	—	—	4.7	36
Total.......................................	13	13	4.7	36
Third-party payment programs:				
Medicare (1966)[e]	69,707	NA	NA	NA
Medicaid (1966)	22,854[f]	NA	NA	NA
Civilian Health and Medical Program of the Uniformed Services (CHAMPUS) (1966)	1,382.7	261.0	156.6	60
NIMH training, research, and prevention programs[g] (1947[h])				
Training..	31.6	31.6	4.8	15
Research:				
Intramural	57.4	57.4	5.5	10
Extramural	98.2	98.2	21.7	22
Biometry and epidemiology	11.5	11.5	2.4	21
Prevention and special mental health	24.1	24.1	10.3	43
Communication and education	2.0	2.0	0.2	10
Total NIMH training, research, and prevention	224.8	224.8	44.9	20

[a]Figures in parentheses indicate fiscal year of program's initiation.
[b]Estimate; States have latitude to transfer limited amounts of funds across program lines.
[c]NA = Not available.
[d]A General Accounting Office survey of 13 States found that States planned to use from none to all of set-aside funds for children's services. See text and table 9.
[e]The Medicare program for enhancing health care to the aged was enacted July 30, 1965, as Title XVIII of the Social Security Act, and expanded to cover the disabled beginning in July 1973, as legislated by the 1972 amendments to the Social Security Act (Public Law 92-603).
[f]In fiscal year 1985, States paid another $18,382 million in Medicaid.
[g]NIMH does not ordinarily aggregate expenditure data by age group; the figures presented here are rough estimates. In addition, NIMH was reorganized in 1985. Program names presented here have changed.
[h]NIMH was created under the Public Health Service Act of 1944 (42 U.S.C. 290 AA-3) and began functioning in late 1947.

SOURCES: **ADM block grant:** R.L. Fogel, "Early Observations on States' Plans To Provide Children's Mental Health Services Under the ADAMH Block Grant (GAO/HRD-85-84)," letter to Senator Inouye from Human Resources Division, General Accounting Office, U.S. Congress, Washington, DC, July 10, 1985. **NIMH:** U.S. Department of Health and Human Services, Public Health Service, National Institute of Mental Health, Alcohol, Drug Abuse, and Mental Health Administration, *Twelfth Annual Report on the Child and Youth Activities of the National Institute of Mental Health, Federal Fiscal Year 1985*, presented to the National Advisory Mental Health Council by M.E. Fishman (Rockville, MD: March 10, 1986). **Medicare:** M. Gornick, J.N. Greenberg, P.. Eggers, and A. Dobson, "Twenty Years of Medicare and Medicaid: Covered Populations, Use of Benefits, and Program Expenditures," *Health Care Financing Review* (1985 Annual Supplement) (Baltimore, MD: U.S. Department of Health and Human Services, Public Health Service, Health Care Financing Administration, December 1985) and Health Care Financing Administration, unpublished data. **Medicaid:** U.S. Department of Health and Human Services, Health Care Financing Administration, Bureau of Program Operations, Grants Branch, Division of State Agency Financial Management, unpublished data pertaining to fiscal year 1985 Medicaid program expenditure information, BPO-F31, Baltimore, MD, September 1986. **CHAMPUS:** K. Zimmerman, Statistics Branch, Information Systems Division, Office of CHAMPUS, personal communication, Sept. 5, 1986.

comparing the treatment costs that each of these sources pays is difficult. In the case of Medicaid, for example, the only mental health expenditure known is that of mental hospitals. Private third-party payers prefer not to disclose what they pay for mental health services, and the amount actually spent by clients themselves is not known.

The proportion of costs specifically for *children's* mental health treatment is even more difficult to determine. It cannot be derived from the proportion of services rendered to children for a number of reasons, perhaps the most important

being that mental health treatment for children is typically more complex and thus more expensive than treatment for adults (see, e.g., 457).

In 1980, an estimated $21 billion was spent by all sources on mental health treatment for all age groups (277a). About half—$10 billion—of this amount was spent for services rendered in the mental health system (277a). (Most of the other expenditures were for treatment rendered in the general health care system.) In 1983, the year closest to 1980 for which data are available, SMHAs reported to the National Association of State

Mental Health Program Directors (NASMHPD) that they spent a total of $6.8 billion on mental health treatment for all age groups (459). This figure allows a rough estimate that more than two-thirds of expenditures for treatment in the mental health system are expenditures made by SMHAs (see figure 4). In turn, most of the revenues to support SMHAs are provided by the States: 76 percent of SMHA revenues in 1983 came from the States, 16 percent from the Federal Government, 3 percent from local governments, and 5 percent from other sources (459).

The NASMHPD study also indicated that SMHAs which were able to determine how much they spent on mental health programs exclusively for children spent an average of 7 percent or about $9 per capita on such programs (459). For adult programs, SMHAs spent an average of 45 percent of their funds, or $22 per capita. These percentages must be viewed with caution, however, because many of the States surveyed could not determine the allocation of mental health funds by age. Further, in all of the States, a substantial portion of mental health funds was spent on programs for all ages combined (e.g., on State mental hospitals).

Alcohol, Drug Abuse, and Mental Health Block Grant

The ADM block grant was initiated in 1981 (Public Law 97-35) as the successor to a variety of categorical programs—most significantly programs under the Community Mental Health Centers Act of 1963 (Public Law 88-164). It is currently the only major Federal program that provides funds to States to support CMHCs and related community mental health services. ADM block grant funds cannot be used for inpatient care.

As shown in table 8, Congress appropriated a total of $490 million for the fiscal year 1985 ADM block grant (considerably less than the $625 million available for categorical programs in fiscal year 1980 (643b)). States receive a share of the ADM total block grant appropriation through a formula based on population and the level of Federal funds received prior to 1981. Because the formula combines population and prior Federal funding levels, there is no direct relationship between the size of the State's population to be served and

Figure 4.—Estimated Proportions of State v. Federal and Private Expenditures for Mental Health Treatment Provided in the Mental Health System to All Age Groups,[a] 1983

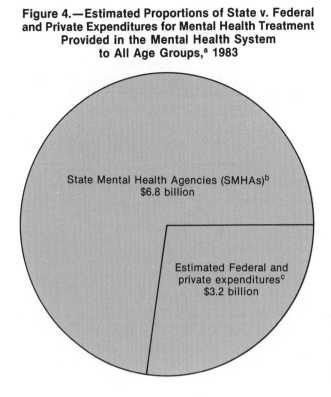

Estimated total: $10 billion

[a]Excludes treatment provided in other service systems (e.g., general health care system).
[b]*Sources of revenue for SMHAs:*
States 76%
Federal Government (e.g., Medicaid [$600 million], Alcohol, Drug Abuse, and Mental Health (ADM) block grant [$200 million]) .16%
Local governments 3%
Other sources 5%
[c]Federal Government share excludes SMHAS (see note b).

SOURCES: **Estimated total:** H. Harwood, D. Napolitano, P. Kristiansen, et al., *Economic Costs to Society of Alcohol and Drug Abuse and Mental Illness: 1980* (Research Triangle Park, NC: Research Triangle Institute, June 1984); **SMHAs:** National Association of State Mental Health Program Directors, *Funding Sources and Expenditures for State Mental Health Agencies: Fiscal Year 1983* (Washington, DC: 1985).

the block grant allocation. Rather the block grant formula tends to "reward" States that relied on Federal funds prior to 1981 and "punish" States that relied to a greater extent on State funds.

For several reasons, it is difficult to determine what portion of ADM block grant funds serves children. First, the ADM block grant is segmented, with separate funding for alcohol, drug abuse, and mental health programs, and the percentage of block grant funds allowed to be used specifically for mental health services differs among States. Second, it is not known to what extent any of the three categories of ADM block grant programs has services designed specifically for children. Third, CMHCs, which receive the bulk of the mental health funds, must provide specialized outpatient services for children, but there is no requirement that they provide a certain level of service or report how much is spent on children's treatment. This situation is different from that under Part F of the Community Mental Health Centers Act of 1963, when specific funds were targeted for children.

In order to better address children's needs, Congress amended the fiscal year 1985 ADM block grant to require that 10 percent of the mental health portion of block grant funds be set aside for "new programs for children and other underserved areas and populations." This set-aside represents a partial return to the Part F targeting policy and reflects a recognition by Congress that children are an underserved population. There was some question, however, as to how effective this 10-percent set-aside would be in increasing the availability of mental health treatment services for children.

To assess the impact of the set-aside, the General Accounting Office (GAO) was requested (by Senator Daniel K. Inouye) to study how States were spending 1985 set-aside funds. Of particular concern was whether set-aside funds were being directed to programs for children and whether these programs were actually "new" programs.

To learn how States were spending 1985 set-aside funds, GAO conducted a telephone survey (during April/May 1985) of 13 States representing each of the Federal regions and approximately 50 percent of the Nation's population (see table 9). Three of the 13 States, Iowa, Mississippi, and Texas, planned to spend all of the 10-percent set-aside moneys on new programs for children. Four of the States, Kentucky, Massachusetts, Michigan, and Washington, had decided not to spend any of the set-aside money on new programs for children. New York had decided that less than one-quarter of its total planned set-aside funds ($203,000 of $1,153,000) would be directed toward new programs for children. Pennsylvania had made a similar decision and allocated approximately 20 percent of its set-aside ($230,000 of $1,325,000) for children's programs. The programs for children to be supported were diverse and included enhancing nonhospital residential care, case management, adolescent problem and suicide prevention, and family support (see table 10).

Table 9.—Fiscal Year 1985 Estimated Allocation of the 10-Percent Set-Aside of the Alcohol, Drug Abuse, and Mental Health (ADM) Block Grant for Selected States (in thousands)[a][b]

State	Total ADM award for fiscal year 1985	Mental health portion of total ADM award amount/percent	Total planned set-aside funds as of May 1985[c]	Set-aside funds allocated for: Children	Underserved areas or populations	Target groups undetermined as of May 1985
California	$48,406	$15,778 (33%)	$2,328	—	—	$2,328
Colorado	7,004	3,400 (49%)	340	$144	$196	0
Florida	24,033	12,855 (53%)	1,358	337	1,021	0
Iowa	2,936	203 (7%)	20	20	0	0
Kentucky	4,551	1,850 (41%)	669	0	669	0
Massachusetts	18,240	10,106 (55%)	1,011	0	1,011	0
Michigan	15,948	4,708 (30%)	471	0	471	0
Mississippi	5,165	3,606 (70%)	361	361	0	0
New York	40,097	9,700 (24%)	1,153	203	950	0
Pennsylvania	25,114	13,250 (53%)	1,326	230	1,096	0
Texas	21,446	8,457 (39%)	846	846	0	0
Vermont	3,313	2,200 (66%)	220	—	—	220
Washington	8,977	4,727 (53%)	526	0	526	0
Total (13 States)	$225,230	$90,840	$10,629	$2,141	$5,940	$2,548

[a]As of May 1985.
[b]Set-aside funds are to be used for new programs only; therefore, amounts in this table do not represent States' entire expenditures on either children or other underserved areas or populations.
[c]Some States set aside more than the required 10 percent of the mental health portion of block grant funds.

SOURCE: R.L. Fogel, "Early Observations on States' Plans To Provide Children's Mental Health Services Under the ADAMH Block Grant (GAO/HRD-85-84)," letter to Senator Inouye from Human Resources Division, General Accounting Office, U.S. Congress, Washington, DC, July 10, 1985.

Table 10.—Planned[a] Use in Selected States of Fiscal Year 1985 Set-Aside Funds for Mental Health Services for Children[b]

State[c]	Services for children
California	Not decided[d]
Colorado	Residential care
Florida	Psychiatric services, summer school session for the handicapped, outpatient, emergency, diagnostic assessment, consultation, case management, crisis intervention, adolescent problem prevention
Iowa	Group home services, adolescent problem prevention, family support
Kentucky	None (funds will be used for other underserved areas or populations)
Massachusetts	None (funds will be used for other underserved areas or populations)
Michigan	None (funds will be used for other underserved areas or populations)
Mississippi	Undetermined[e]
New York	Family support, adolescent suicide prevention, referral
Pennsylvania	Residential care
Texas	Services for students with drug or alcohol problems, weapons violations, etc., services for minority inhalant abusers
Vermont	Not decided[d]
Washington	None (funds will be used for other underserved areas or populations)

[a]As of May 1985.

[b]Block grant set-aside funds were also permitted to be used for underserved populations other than children. In addition, some underserved populations that the States reported were to be served (e.g., the homeless chronically mentally ill) were not targeted by age. Some of these programs may address the mental health needs of children.

[c]A sample of 13 States, representing the receipt of about half the Alcohol, Drug Abuse, and Mental Health block grant funds, were surveyed by the General Accounting Office.

[d]"Not decided" indicates that the State had not decided whether set-aside funds were to be used for children or for other underserved areas or populations.

[e]"Undetermined" indicates that the State had decided to use set-aside funds for children and adolescents, but had not decided which services the funds were to be used for.

SOURCE: R.L. Fogel, "Early Observations on States' Plans To Provide Children's Mental Health Services Under the ADAMH Block Grant (GAO/HRD-85-84)," letter to Senator Inouye from Human Resources Division, General Accounting Office, U.S. Congress, Washington, DC, July 10, 1985.

It is important to emphasize that the entire ADM block grant is small in comparison to State funds and that the 10-percent set-aside for children and other underserved populations is taken only from the mental health portion of the ADM block grant. The entire 10-percent set-aside may be less than $20 million nationwide—and only a portion of this would be directed to new programs for children. Because there were no new funds, the set-aside requirements might mean that funds for new programs for children will have to be taken from other existing programs, unless States make up the funds for other programs. Some

States noted that the requirement that the programs for children or other underserved populations be "new" did not allow for additional funds to be allocated to already existing programs that appeared to be effective. In response to these problems, Congress amended the 10 percent set-aside in fiscal year 1986 to read that 10-percent of mental health block grant funds could be used for "new or expanded" programs for underserved populations, with a "special emphasis" on children or adolescents (Public Law 99-117).

Perhaps the most important impact of the set-aside is symbolic. As States are required to report the amounts of ADM block grant money spent on new programs for children, more attention may be brought to children's mental health problems. Also, because funds from the ADM block grant cannot be spent on inpatient services, the program provides an incentive for States to develop locally based outpatient treatment programs. To the extent that resources for outpatient programs are available, early diagnosis and treatment for children with mental health problems may be more likely.

Federal Third-Party Payment Programs

The Federal Government plays a major and trend-setting role in financing health care services. It is the largest single insurer of health care services (Medicare and partial funding of Medicaid) and has also played a leadership role in the development of health care payment systems. The extent to which certain services and providers receive reimbursement while others do not has a direct effect on the delivery of care (206). Traditionally, coverage for mental health services has been less extensive than coverage for other medical services (e.g., see 20,175a). Mental health coverage is also limited by requirements for the presence of a diagnosable disorder (see ch. 3) as a condition for reimbursement.

Three key parts of the Federal health care financing system are Medicaid, Medicare, and CHAMPUS. In 1985, Medicaid served 11 million (296,297) dependent children under the age of 21, but the amount of mental health benefits provided to these children is believed to be minimal. Medicare provides no significant funding for children's mental health care, but Medicaid and other third-party payers that do fund such care are often influenced by Medicare's payment policies. CHAMPUS is the largest single health insurance program in the country, providing coverage for health services to military dependents and retirees who are unable to receive services through uniformed service medical treatment facilities. CHAMPUS spends 60 percent of its mental health expenditures on treatment for children.

Medicaid.—Medicaid represents 55 percent of all public health funds spent on children (645) and has the potential to meet the needs of children who are possibly at the greatest risk for developing mental disorders, those who are in poverty and those who are uninsured.

In general, Medicaid provides health insurance to low-income families who meet certain categorical and financial criteria. These criteria, and many of the services provided, are generally set by the States, which provide a very significant portion of the Medicaid funding. Medicaid serves approximately 11 million children. Most important for purposes of this background paper is that while beneficiaries may not be discriminated against on the basis of diagnosis, States are free to set limitations on Medicaid coverage for mental health services (636). The percentage of Medicaid funds devoted to mental health care is not known. GAO is conducting a national survey of the mental health services available under Medicaid.

Medicaid's Early and Periodic Screening, Diagnosis, and Treatment (EPSDT) program provides funds to screen, diagnose, and treat children under 21 who are members of families designated as "categorically needy," and so is a potentially important Federal initiative (434). The developmental assessment that is required as part of EPSDT screening can reveal emotional difficulties and problems in behavior development. However, because of changes in eligibility, children may not be followed long enough for a developmental assessment to be adequate; in addition, few States deliver any substantial amount of mental health care through this program (358,595).

Efforts in the late 1970s to upgrade EPSDT into a Child Health Assurance Program (CHAP), and thus to specifically require mental health assessment and treatment for Medicaid-eligible children, were not successful (595). An expansion of Medicaid eligibility passed in 1984 (Public Law 98-369) is potentially important for preventing, detecting, and treating mental health problems because it makes additional women and children eligible for medical services. Although this expansion of eligibility is sometimes referred to as a "modified CHAP," it did not specifically require mental health assessment and treatment for children.

In addition to the expansion of eligibility, another potentially important change in the Medicaid program was incorporated in the Consolidated Omnibus Budget Reconciliation Act (COBRA) of 1985 (Public Law 99-272), which was signed into law on April 7, 1986. Under the provisions of COBRA, States will be allowed to cover case management services, which were defined as those services that assist individuals eligible under Medicaid to gain access to needed medical, social, educational, and other services.

It appears that Medicaid may ensure that at least some poor people obtain mental health care who would not otherwise do so. An analysis by Taube and Rupp (632a) found that poor and near-poor Medicaid recipients were more likely than nonrecipients to get mental health treatment. As noted above, States have different Medicaid eligibility requirements, so Taube and Rupp were able to compare persons who were of similar socioeconomic status. Taube and Rupp attribute the greater use of mental health benefits by Medicaid recipients to the fact that Medicaid does not allow cost-sharing (i.e., recipients are not required to pay any of the costs of health services). Taube and Rupp's finding, as well as their interpretation, is consistent with other studies which show that the use of mental health care is responsive to the cost of such care, although cost is not the only factor which determines whether people seek mental health care (206).

Medicare.—The Medicare program covers the cost of hospitalization, medical care, and related services for most persons over age 65, persons receiving social security disability insurance payments for 2 years, and persons with end-stage renal disease. Although only a small proportion of Medicare program funds are directly devoted to children (children who are disabled and dependents of deceased, retired, or disabled social security beneficiaries), Medicare influences health care reimbursement nationwide. Not only have a number of States adopted Medicare rules for payment of Medicaid and other insurance benefits, but non-Federal health insurance providers closely watch Medicare.

The Social Security Amendments of 1983 (Public Law 98-21) mandated that Medicare adopt a prospective payment system[1] for hospitals (648, 649). Children's hospitals and psychiatric hospitals, along with rehabilitation and long-term care hospitals, have been temporarily exempted from the new payment system; however, the system does apply to psychiatric services provided in nonspecialized units in general hospitals.

Medicare's prospective payment system is based on fixed per-case payment rates for patients in 467 diagnosis-related groups (DRGs). DRGs are a patient classification system developed at Yale for purposes of research on health care delivery. There are nine DRGs for "mental diseases" and six for substance abuse (see table 11).

DRG 431, "childhood mental disorders," includes diagnoses of childhood-onset mental disorders (see ch. 3). Because many childhood diagnoses can also be applied to adults (e.g., a problem such as attention deficit disorder, which has its onset in childhood), DRG 431 does not apply only to children. Furthermore, DRG 431 is not the only DRG applied to children with mental disorders. Children with mental disorders that can also receive an adult diagnosis (e.g., adolescents with drug or alcohol abuse problems) are sometimes placed in other categories. Nonetheless, DRG 431 is probably the most frequently used DRG for children, and so deserves careful attention in the event a prospective payment system is considered for the children's mental health care system.

Like most DRGs, DRG 431 does not differentiate patient episodes by problem severity, treatment modality and setting, or the patient's history. The Medicare payment rate for DRG 431 is based on an adjusted average (the geometric mean[2]) of lengths of stay (LOS) in the hospital among patients with this diagnosis. In the case of DRG 431, this equals 15.4 days. As indicated in table 11, however, DRG 431 is the mental disorder DRG category with the most variation in LOS (632), with few patients being treated close to the 15.4-day mean LOS. Approximately 25 percent of patients in DRG 431 have an LOS less than 10 days, while 25 percent have an LOS greater than 75 days. Since DRG-based payment by Medicare does not take LOS into account, a hospital treating an individual with a childhood-onset mental disorder for 75 days receives the same Medicare payment as a hospital treating the individual for 1 day or for 15.4 days.

Variation in LOS for DRG 431 aside, there are a number of potentially serious problems connected with application of a DRG-based payment system to children's mental health care (581). One basic problem is that there is no theoretical or empirical evidence to indicate that the use of treatment resources is related to a mentally disturbed child's diagnosis. Systems of classifying mental disorders (such as the American Psychiatric Association's *Diagnostic and Statistical Manual* or the World Health Organization's *International Classification of Diseases*) indicate only the related set of conditions that have been found for a particular syndrome. These systems were not designed to be used for reimbursement purposes (19) and do not necessarily indicate the severity of a mental disturbance. Especially for children, mental health treatment decisions may be based on the family's ability to manage the child as well as on the multiplicity of problems faced by the child.

In the absence of a direct relationship between diagnosis and length/intensity/cost of mental health treatment, DRG-based payment will not be likely to match a child's need for services. In the short term, a mismatch between DRG-based payment and the cost of needed services may result in some (probably the most troubled) children's being denied services. It may also result in

---

[1]Prospective payment, payment to health care providers based on rates established in advance, is an alternative to retrospective cost-based reimbursement, under which payment to providers is based on the amount and type of services they provide (648,707).

[2]Like the arithmetic mean, or average, the geometric mean is a central value in a distribution of scores that serves as a summary measure of the scores. By relying on logarithms, the geometric mean has the advantage of being less influenced by the uneven distribution of scores.

Table 11.—Lengths of Stay Associated With Mental Disorder Diagnosis-Related Groups (DRGs) Ranked by Interquartile Range

DRG	Length of stay in days			
	Geometric mean[a]	25th percentile	75th percentile	Interquartile range[b] (75th percentile minus 25th percentile
Childhood mental disorders (431).....................	15.4	9.8	75.5	65.0
Organic disturbances and mental retardation (429).......	8.8	9.2	34.4	25.0
Psychoses (430)..	10.8	8.7	32.7	24.0
Alcohol dependence (436)	8.1	4.8	26.9	22.0
Disorders of personality and impulse control (428).......	8.3	4.8	25.5	20.0
Depressive neuroses (426)............................	9.4	6.1	25.3	19.0
Drug dependence (434)...............................	9.1	6.9	25.5	18.0
Neuroses except depressive (427)	6.9	4.8	22.4	17.0
Other mental disorder diagnoses (432)	7.2	7.7	23.0	15.0
Drug use except dependence (435)	8.0	4.2	19.4	15.0
Acute adjustment reaction/disturbances of psychosocial dysfunction (425)	5.8	3.3	18.3	15.0
Alcohol use except dependence (437).................	3.5	3.1	14.8	11.0
Alcohol- and substance-induced organic mental syndrome (438)......................................	6.9	3.9	15.5	11.0
Substance use and substance-induced organic mental disorder, left against medical advice (433)	2.5	1.9	9.6	7.0

[a]Like the arithmetic mean, or average, the geometric mean is a central value in a distribution of scores that serves as a summary measure of the scores. By relying on logarithms, the geometric mean has the advantage of being less influenced by the uneven distribution of scores.
[b]The interquartile range is the range of scores extending equally on both sides of the mean that covers the middle 50 percent of a distribution of scores. Thus, the interquartile range is a measure of variation, in this instance, in length of stay.

SOURCE: From C. Taube, E.S. Lee, and R.N. Forthofer, "Diagnosis-Related Groups for Mental Disorders, Alcoholism, and Drug Abuse: Evaluation and Alternatives," *Hospital and Community Psychiatry* 35(5):453-454, 1984.

unnecessary and inappropriate treatment as hospitals are provided an incentive to treat "simple" cases. The long-term impact on the range and quality of available services is unknown (649).

A second critical problem with the application of a DRG-based payment system to children's mental health care is that the data used to calculate average LOS, on which DRG payment is based, were derived from past experience in a sample of adult acute care hospitals. Data reflecting the types of treatments given to children in specialized psychiatric units or in psychiatric hospitals were not included.

Even if LOS data were available from hospital facilities that treat mentally disturbed children, however, there would be a serious problem in using such data. Most health benefit programs have limitations on the type and amount of both inpatient and outpatient treatment provided. In addition, most benefit programs provide more generous coverage for inpatient care than for outpatient, residential treatment center (RTC), or day treatment (600).

The fundamental problem with application of a DRG-based payment system to children's mental health services is that basing payment on a broad category of diagnosis such as "childhood mental disorders" ignores the body of literature on the variety of treatment needs of mentally disturbed children. This problem exists for other DRGs and other vulnerable populations as well (649). A DRG-based prospective payment system may control costs and maintain quality of care for patients who require specific medical or surgical procedures (i.e., non-mental-health care), but it seems inappropriate and potentially harmful to apply such a DRG-based payment system to children's mental health care.

Civilian Health and Medical Program of the Uniformed Services.—CHAMPUS is a health insurance program administered by the U.S. Department of Defense (DOD). CHAMPUS provides health benefits to 6.5 million military dependents and retirees who are unable to receive services through uniformed service medical treatment facilities, and is known as one of the most generous third-party payers for mental health care.

Primarily because few uniformed service medical treatment facilities offer mental health services, CHAMPUS devotes a higher percentage of its benefit payments (16 to 19 percent [643a,655]; also see table 8) to mental health services than do most private insurance plans. Another reason that CHAMPUS devotes a high percentage of its benefit payments to mental health services is that military families often live in areas not adequately served by outpatient mental health professionals; for families in areas not served by outpatient facilities, the only mental health treatment option may be psychiatric hospitalization, or, for children, care in an RTC. Inpatient and RTC treatment are typically more expensive than outpatient treatment; and CHAMPUS spends up to 75 percent of its mental health benefits on inpatient and RTC treatment (548), despite the presence of an unusually rigorous peer review system which must certify all care (inpatient, outpatient, residential) as medically or psychologically necessary (548, 549).

In their efforts to control the costs of mental health care under CHAMPUS, both Congress and CHAMPUS have implemented provisions for maximum benefits for mental health care in psychiatric hospitals and, more recently, in RTCs. The effect of one such provision—a 60-day "cap" on inpatient psychiatric hospitalization—illustrates how changes in reimbursement policy can change the type of services available. This example is not definitive, however, because the change in CHAMPUS reimbursement policy was not introduced experimentally (i.e., with use of a control group experiencing no changes in coverage). Thus, alternative explanations for subsequent variations in treatment services, such as changes in treatment philosophy, cannot be ruled out.

Under the 60-day cap, exceptional justification of medical necessity has to be provided for psychiatric hospitalization longer than 60 days for both adults and children or CHAMPUS will not pay for the care. Extension of the 60-day limit is granted only if a patient is a danger to himself/herself or others; or if the patient has a medical complication and only an inpatient hospital facility can provide appropriate treatment. The cap does not affect RTCs.

A 1985 DOD analysis of the first year's experience with the 60-day cap concluded that the 60-day limit on inpatient psychiatric hospitalization had resulted in a $34.2 million "cost avoidance," representing 22 percent of the total CHAMPUS spent for inpatient and RTC mental health care in calendar year 1983 (655). Perhaps as expected, there was a 66-percent increase in RTC admissions in 1983, although the costs of RTC stays were not included in DOD's analysis (655). The cost of inpatient care cannot be separated from the costs of RTC care in CHAMPUS's data system. DOD's analysis was adjusted, however, for an estimated 80,000 outpatient visits attributed to the 60-day cap.

On the basis of its 1985 analysis and subsequent monitoring, CHAMPUS more recently estimated that there would be a 100-percent increase in admissions to RTCs between 1983 and 1986 (from 425 in 1983 to about 850 in 1986 [643a]). In addition, CHAMPUS reported that since the imposition of the 60-day cap, there had been an increase in the number of RTCs attached to psychiatric hospitals that had applied and been approved under CHAMPUS (from 13 in December 1982 to 30 in December 1985 [643a]). In order to provide additional long-term control over cost escalation, CHAMPUS has since developed a new policy to limit its payments for RTC care.

As do all health care cost-containment efforts, CHAMPUS's attempts to limit costs raise concerns about maintaining good quality care. CHAMPUS monitors quality through its unusually rigorous peer review system and its approval processes (548, 549). In addition, GAO is studying methods for assessing the quality of care provided under CHAMPUS.

The Education for All Handicapped Children Act (Public Law 94-142)

The Education for All Handicapped Children Act (Public Law 94-142) mandates that all physically and mentally handicapped children be provided a free, appropriate education and the "related services" necessary to obtain an education (see ch. 7). The Federal Government provides a small amount of grant money to States to help them implement this law.

There is continuing debate about whether mental health care is properly included under "related services." Even those who consider mental health interventions necessary for education disagree about where the responsibility for payment lies—with the school system, the welfare system, the health care system, or the mental health care system. There is additional concern about the costs and personnel required when residential treatment is indicated, and about whether the school systems should be required to pay for the entire costs of residential placements or only for the education-related costs (109). Evidence suggests that the services available to mentally disturbed children through Public Law 94-142 vary considerably by State (657). When this background paper was being written, a study was being conducted to determine what related services, including mental health services, were being provided under Public Law 94-142 (666).

Coordination of Services

The State Comprehensive Mental Health Services Plan Act of 1986 (Public Law 99-660)

In response to the perceived inadequacy and fragmentation of services for individuals who are perhaps most in need of coordinated mental health and other system services—the chronically mentally ill, Congress has passed legislation to encourage a continuum of services and coordination among agencies. The most recent legislation in this vein is Public Law 99-660, the State Comprehensive Mental Health Services Plan Act of 1986, passed in November 1986. This law authorizes a total of $20 million in grants to States for fiscal years 1987 and 1988 for the development of State comprehensive mental health services plans and provides direction on the content of such plans. Perhaps most significant, State plans are required to provide for the establishment and implementation of organized community-based systems of care for chronically mentally ill individuals; and to require the provision of case management to each chronically mentally ill individual. The law also expands the focus of the already existing Federal Community Support Program (in NIMH) to include the homeless chronically mentally ill.

It is too early to tell, of course, how States will respond to the new grant program or to what extent the program will affect children. An earlier program to encourage the integration of mental health and other services for children, CASSP, was, as is described below, enthusiastically responded to by States. Neither the new program nor CASSP, however, address the needs of children with mental health problems that are not yet severe or chronic. The analysis in this background paper, like analyses of past national commissions, suggests that the needs of such children are urgent.

Child and Adolescent Service System Program

CASSP, administered by NIMH, is a direct response to the lack of coordination among the settings and systems providing services to children with mental health problems. Modeled after the Community Support Program for the chronically mentally ill, CASSP was created by Congress in 1984 after repeated findings that because of a lack of coordination among systems of care, the individual programs designed to assist mentally disturbed children were frequently not used. The goal of CASSP is to ensure the availability of a comprehensive, coordinated system of care specifically for severely mentally disturbed children and adolescents.

Several themes developed earlier in this background paper point to the need for coordinating mental health and other children's services. Disturbed children often have more than one mental health problem (e.g., an attention deficit and reading disorder that become apparent in school combined with aggressive behavior in the neighborhood). Many troubled children also have educational, physical, legal, economic, or family problems in addition to their mental disturbance. Given the interactions among disturbed children's problems, effective intervention often requires the provision of a variety of multiple mental health and other services. CASSP was based on the belief that coordination among mental health treatment and other service systems is necessary to ensure that severely disturbed children receive all the services they need, organized into a comprehensive treatment plan, and timed to achieve optimal beneficial effects.

CASSP is designed to improve States' capacities to offer aid to severely mentally disturbed children. CASSP assists States in developing systems of care through planning grants, as well as technical assistance and training. States that receive CASSP grants are required, initially, to develop a child mental health authority and to organize a "coalition" of State agencies whose work affects children. Once a comprehensive State-level system is developed, the goal is to replicate the coordination effort at local levels.

It is too early to assess the effectiveness of the CASSP grant program, but the program incorporates a number of elements of an ideal system that have long been discussed. By focusing on the organization of services, it advances the goals of placing children in appropriate settings and having providers make treatment decisions based on clinical needs rather than on maintaining fiscal solvency. CASSP is designed to help States develop mechanisms which may differ across localities and available resources, and it appears to be an important mechanism to facilitate development of such locally controlled systems of care. As described in chapter 9 of this background paper, State authorities and NIMH are jointly developing an evaluation of CASSP's effects.

Research and Training

For research related to children's mental health and for training clinical and research professionals in this area, the Federal Government is virtually the only source of funds. With few exceptions, such as the MacArthur Foundation, neither philanthropic foundations nor individual donors support research or training in the mental health field (309). SMHAs spend very little on research and training. Some critics charge that the funds available to support mental health research are inadequate to take advantage of "exciting" research opportunities or even to foster rational development of the field (309). Research on childhood mental disorders is frequently used as a prime example of the opportunities that are missed.

Funds for research pertaining to children's mental health are available primarily through NIMH. NIMH research grants are available for a range of disciplines, including behavioral science research, clinical research, the neurosciences, pharmacological and somatic treatments, and psychosocial treatments. As shown in table 8, NIMH estimates that roughly $27.2 million was made available in fiscal year 1985 for intramural and extramural research relating to children's mental health (665). This amount represents 17 percent of NIMH's research budget (see table 8).

The main direct source of funds for training mental health professionals to treat children is the clinical training program of NIMH. Since 1983, congressional appropriations committees have requested that NIMH allocate a portion of its clinical training funds specifically to mental health professionals who treat underserved populations, including children. Because NIMH has limited funds overall and commitments to continue existing training grants, however, the impact on children's mental health services has only begun to be seen.

In fiscal year 1985, NIMH allocated approximately 15 percent of its clinical training funds, or $4.8 million, to training programs dealing at least in part with children's mental health issues (see table 8).

A major reason for targeting NIMH clinical training funds to professionals who treat children is that there appear to be insufficient numbers of well-trained professionals to meet children's needs. According to 1976 data (109), only 10 percent of psychiatrists are specifically trained to treat children, and less than 1 percent of psychologists primarily serve children. According to NIMH data, there are approximately 3,000 child psychiatrists, 5,000 clinical child psychologists, 7,000 child and family-oriented social workers, and 1,000 child/family-oriented mental health nurses (358). Estimates of the numbers of professionals needed have consistently been much higher.

Funds for training mental health researchers (as opposed to clinicians) are available through NIMH under authority of the National Research Services Awards Act (Public Law 93-348). Although the Institute of Medicine (309) has called for increased funding of research training in children's mental health, calling this a "relatively unstudied area," only $1.1 million for training researchers was available through NIMH in fiscal year 1984 (664).

Information about the mental health training funds available from agencies other than NIMH is less clear. The Education for All Handicapped Children Act (Public Law 94-142) includes Federal funding for training special education personnel, but this training is directed at all handicapping conditions covered under the law. Although it is certain that funds could be well used for professional development in child welfare, juvenile justice, and education agencies to promote the integration of mental health services with these related services, there are currently no major Federal programs to support this kind of integrative training.

Prevention and Other Services

A number of Federal programs provide funds that may be used to support delivery of mental health treatment or that have a clearly positive or preventive role in children's mental health. These include the programs that primarily provide health services, as well as those providing social services, nutrition assistance, and direct or indirect financial payments.

The Maternal and Child Health block grant is a Federal program that provides funds to the States for services to mothers and children, particularly in low-income families. Since adequate health care is vital for promoting normal and healthy development in children, these block grant funds can play a significant role in the prevention of mental illness in children. Medical care providers who treat children who have no link with mental health care providers through the schools or other agencies are often the first to identify emotional or psychological problems that may require treatment (see ch. 7).

A Federal program related to the Maternal and Child Health block grant, the Primary Care block grant, gives Federal funds directly to community health centers for general health care services to medically underserved populations. These general health care services provide a measure of prevention and screening for mental health problems affecting children and their families, and provide a point of contact with health care providers. Similarly, the Preventive Health and Health Services block grant provides Federal funds to States for a variety of preventive health programs, including home health services, rape prevention and treatment services, and demonstration projects specifically designed to deter consumption of alcohol among children and adolescents. Many of these programs serve an important prevention function for mental disorders.

Three other major Federal support programs have important effects on children's mental health. The Title XX Social Services block grant provides funds to States for a wide variety of social services to children and families, including day care, protective services for children, family planning, adoption, and foster care. These services have played a major role in the promotion of child welfare. The Adoption Assistance and Child Welfare Act (Public Law 96-272) funds child welfare services, foster care, adoption assistance for hard-to-place children (including those who are emotionally or intellectually handicapped), and has, in general, been helpful in financing support services to aid children and families in crisis. Project Head Start provides educational, social, health, and nutrition services to low-income preschool children. The long-term effectiveness of Head Start programs in preventing problems is now well recognized (728; also see ch. 9).

Among the other Federal programs that relate to children's mental health, directly or indirectly, are funding programs designed to enable individuals to meet basic health, nutrition, and cost-of-living needs. Such programs include the Child Abuse Prevention and Treatment Act programs; Victims of Crime Act programs; Developmental Disabilities Assistance and Bill of Rights Act programs; Family Planning programs; the Foster Grandparents Program; the Adolescent Family Life Program; the Food Stamp Program; the Supplemental Food Program for Women, Infants, and Children; School Lunch programs; Aid to Families with Dependent Children; Supplemental Security Income; Child Support Enforcement programs; and income tax deductions for adopting special-needs children. As part of the overall Federal effort relevant to children's mental health, these programs provide a considerable amount of assistance. It is not clear, however, that the assistance provided by these programs is coordinated so that individual children are protected. Previous analyses (e.g., 358,595), anecdotal evidence, and observations of the experts consulted during the preparation of this background paper suggest that a coordinated system for providing children's services would be helpful. Perhaps the evaluation of CASSP and experience under the State Comprehensive Mental Health Services Plan Act will suggest additional ways in which such coordination can be implemented.

CONCLUSION

It is quite well established that a great many children are in need of mental health services—both to treat diagnosable disorders and to reduce environmental risk factors (see ch. 2). It is also agreed that children's mental health services need to be based on extensive and sound research; guided by appropriately trained personnel; and supported by sufficient funds and incentives to encourage coordination among providers, including those in non-mental-health systems.

Federal, State, local, and private contributions to provision of mental health services are substantial. The gap between the need for children's services and the availability of such services, however, implies that even these considerable efforts fall short of bridging the gap (e.g., 358,359). The mental health services available for children appear to be inadequate. In addition, research on children's mental health and illness appears to be inadequately funded.

Although local control of service delivery is believed to be optimal for the necessary case management of children with problems and potential problems, and although the private sector could arrange to provide more and better mental health services, it may be that a larger role for the Federal Government is desirable. Such a role could include a statement of principle for mental health analogous to that articulated for education in Public Law 94-142, which mandates that all children be guaranteed a free, appropriate education. It could also include increased Federal efforts to eradicate environmental risk factors or reduce

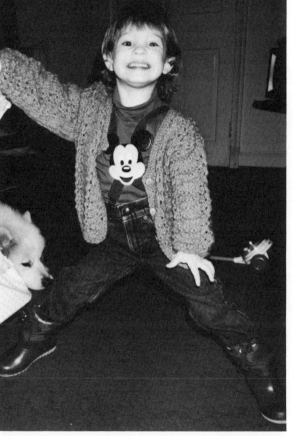

Photo credit: OTA

their impact on children, to continue to promote coordination of services, and to fund research and training in the children's mental health field.

Appendixes

Workshop Participants and Other Acknowledgments

Workshop on Children's Mental Health

Leonore Behar, *Chair*
Chief of Child Mental Health Services, North Carolina Department of Human Resources
Division of Mental Health, Mental Retardation, and Substance Abuse Services
Raleigh, NC

Mark Blotcky
Timberlawn Hospital
Dallas, TX

Dennis D. Drotar
Rainbow Babies and Children's Hospital
Cleveland, OH

Susan Goldstein
Department of Child and Family Psychiatry
Group Health Association
Washington, DC

Erv Janssen
Director, Children's Division
Menninger Foundation
Topeka, KS

Hubert E. Jones
Dean, School of Social Work
Boston University
Boston, MA

Patricia King
Professor
Georgetown Law Center
Washington, DC

Jane Knitzer
Director, Division of Research, Demonstrations,
   and Policy[1]
Bank Street College of Education
New York, NY

Gerald P. Koocher
Department of Psychiatry
Children's Hospital Medical Center
Boston, MA

Judith Meyers
Policy Analyst[2]
Office of the Governor
Boston, MA

Joseph J. Palombi
Family Counseling Center
Fairfax, VA

Patricia C. Pothier
Professor
University of California, School of Nursing
San Francisco, CA

Jack Shonkoff
Department of Pediatrics
University of Massachusetts
Worcester, MA

Jerry Wiener
Chairman
Department of Psychiatry
George Washington University Medical School
Washington, DC

Edward Zigler
Department of Psychology
Yale University
New Haven, CT

NIMH Liaison

Michael Fishman
Assistant Director for Children and Youth
National Institute of Mental Health
Rockville, MD

---

[1]Formerly with the Bunting Institute, Radcliffe College, Cambridge, MA.
[2]Formerly Associate Director, Bush Program in Child Development and Social Policy, University of Michigan, Ann Arbor, MI.

Workshop on Children's Mental Health Treatment Effectiveness

Anthony Broskowski
Executive Director
Northside Community Mental Health Center
Tampa, FL

Donald Cohen
Director, Child Study Center
Yale University
New Haven, CT

John P. Docherty
Chief, Psychosocial Treatments Research Branch[1]
National Institute of Mental Health
Rockville, MD

Michael E. Fishman
Associate Director for Children and Youth
National Institute of Mental Health
Rockville, MD

Alan E. Kazdin
Professor of Psychiatry and Psychology
Western Psychiatric Institute and Clinic
Pittsburgh, PA

Ira Lourie
Director, Child and Adolescent Service System
    Program
National Institute of Mental Health
Rockville, MD

Natalie Reatig
Pharmacologic and Somatic Treatments Research
    Branch
National Institute of Mental Health
Rockville, MD

---

[1]No longer with NIMH.

Acknowledgments

OTA would like to thank the following people for their assistance in the development of this background paper.

Richard Brunstetter
National Institute of Mental Health
Rockville, MD

Lana Buck
National Association of Private Psychiatric
    Hospitals
Washington, DC

Barbara Burns
National Institute of Mental Health
Rockville, MD

Anne Copeland
Boston University
Boston, MA

Mary Crosby
American Academy of Child and Adolescent
    Psychiatry
Washington, DC

Phyllis Old Dog Cross
Indian Health Service
Rapid City, SD

Felton Earls
Washington University School of Medicine
St. Louis, MO

Glen Elliott
Stanford University
Stanford, CA

Michelle Fine
University of Pennsylvania
Philadelphia, PA

Judith Gardner
Boston, MA

Ellen Greenberg Garrison
American Psychological Association
Washington, DC

Howard Goldman
National Institute of Mental Health
Rockville, MD

Dennis C. Harper
University of Iowa
Iowa City, IA

Victor Indrisano
Office of U.S. Rep. Edward R. Roybal
Washington, DC

Joseph Jacobs
Bureau of Health Care Delivery and Assistance
U.S. Public Health Service
Rockville, MD

Judith Jacobs
National Institute of Mental Health
Rockville, MD

Phyllis A. Katz
Institute for Research on Social Problems
Boulder, CO

Judith Katz-Leavy
National Institute of Mental Health
Rockville, MD

Samuel C. Klagsbrun
Four Winds Hospital
Katohah, NY

Lt. Col. Melvin Kolb
Office of the Civilian Health and Medical Program
  of the Uniformed Services
Aurora, CO

Richard Krugman
National Center for Child Abuse
Denver, CO

Sidney S. Lee
Milbank Memorial Fund
New York, NY

Beryce W. MacLennan
U.S. General Accounting Office
Washington, DC

Noel Mazade
Noel Mazade & Associates, Inc.
Garrett Park, MD

Irving Philips
University of California
San Francisco, CA

Cornelia Porter
Office of Senator Daniel K. Inouye
Washington, DC

Paul Posner
U.S. General Accounting Office
Washington, DC

Lenore Radloff
National Institute of Mental Health
Rockville, MD

Mason Russell
Policy Analysis
Brookline, MA

Jack Sarmanian
Adult/Adolescent Counseling, Inc.
Malden, MA

Larry Silver
National Institute of Mental Health
Rockville, MD

Morton Silverman
National Institute of Mental Health
Rockville, MD

Carl R. Smith
Iowa Department of Public Instruction
Des Moines, IA

Albert J. Solnit
Yale University
New Haven, CT

Fredric Solomon
Institute of Medicine
Washington, DC

Brian Stabler
American Psychological Association
Washington, DC

Bonnie Strickland
University of Massachusetts
Amherst, MA

Susan Thompson-Hoffman
U.S. Department of Education
Washington, DC

Carl Tishler
Columbus, OH

Gail Toff
Intergovernmental Health Policy Project
Washington, DC

Judith L. Wagner
Office of Technology Assessment
Washington, DC

Ted Wagner
U.S. General Accounting Office
Washington, DC

Kathleen Wells
Bellefaire
Cleveland, OH

Diana Zuckerman
Subcommittee on Intergovernmental Relations and
  Human Resources
House Government Operations Committee
Washington, DC

List of Acronyms and Glossary of Terms

List of Acronyms

ADAMHA	—Alcohol, Drug Abuse, and Mental Health Administration (DHHS)
ADM	—Alcohol, Drug Abuse, and Mental Health (block grant)
CASSP	—Child and Adolescent Service System Program (NIMH)
CDF	—Children's Defense Fund
CHAMPUS	—Civilian Health and Medical Program of the Uniformed Services
CMHC	—community mental health center
COBRA	—Consolidated Omnibus Budget Reconciliation Act
DHEW	—U.S. Department of Health, Education, and Welfare (now DHHS)
DHHS	—U.S. Department of Health and Human Services
DISC	—Diagnostic Interview Schedule for Children
DOD	—U.S. Department of Defense
DRG	—diagnosis-related group
DSM-III	—*Diagnostic and Statistical Manual*, 3rd ed.
EPSDT	—Early and Periodic Screening, Diagnosis, and Treatment program (Medicaid)
FSCP	—Family Support Center Program
GAO	—General Accounting Office (U.S. Congress)
LOS	—length of stay
NASMHPD	—National Association of State Mental Health Program Directors
NIMH	—National Institute of Mental Health (ADAMHA)
OTA	—Office of Technology Assessment (U.S. Congress)
PDD	—pervasive developmental disorder
RTC	—residential treatment center for emotionally disturbed children
SDD	—specific developmental disorder
SMHA	—State Mental Health Agency

Glossary of Terms

Adjustment disorder: A type of mental disorder defined by DSM-III as "a maladaptive reaction to an identifiable psychosocial stressor that occurs within three months of the onset of the stressor." Adjustment disorders are manifest in impaired functioning or in excessive reactions to the stressor, symptoms which typically remit after the stressor ceases or, if the stressor continues, when a new level of adaptive functioning is achieved.

Aftercare: Mental health services provided after the individual's initial encounter with the mental health care system (e.g., RTC treatment after psychiatric hospitalization).

Anorexia nervosa: A mental disorder characterized by intense fear of becoming obese, disturbance of body image, significant weight loss (accounted for by no known physical disorder), refusal to maintain a minimal normal body weight, and the absence of menstruation in females.

Anxiety disorders: A category of mental health disorders characterized by a child's intense feelings of apprehension, tension, or uneasiness. These feelings may result from the anticipation of danger, either internal or external. Anxiety is manifested by physiological changes such as sweating, tremor, and rapid pulse. Such disorders include phobic disorders, obsessive compulsive disorders, and post-traumatic stress disorders, as well as "generalized anxiety disorders."

Behavior disorders: A set of childhood-onset mental disorders characterized by behavior that disturbs or harms the patient or others and which causes distress or disability. Such disorders include attention deficit disorder and conduct disorder.

Behavioral therapy: Psychotherapy based on the assumption that a child learns persistent pathological behavior from his or her experience with the social environment. Therapists using behavioral techniques systematically analyze the child's problem and environment and seek to change specific problem behavior by altering the child's environment.

Bulimia: A mental disorder characterized by binge eating accompanied by an awareness that the eating pattern is abnormal, fear of not being able to stop eating voluntarily, and depressed mood and self-deprecating thoughts following the eating binges. Binges are usually terminated temporarily by abdominal pain, sleep, social interruption, or induced vomiting.

Cognitive therapy: Psychotherapy based on a view that mental health problems should be treated through altering the way children think about their behavior and their environments. Therapists attempt to change the thinking that takes place during a child's troublesome behavior and/or try to influence how children think about themselves and others.

Community mental health centers (CMHCs): Programs initially established by the Federal Government through the Community Mental Health Centers Act of 1963, to provide comprehensive mental health services to all residents of a specified geographic area regardless of their ability to pay. With the passage of the Alcohol, Drug Abuse, and Mental Health block grant, federally funded CMHCs ceased to exist as legal entities, but Federal funds continue to be provided indirectly via State Mental Health Agencies.

Continuum of care: A coordinated system to provide comprehensive children's mental health care at all levels needed.

Day treatment/partial hospitalization: Mental health treatment programs that provide extended care to children who do not need 24-hour treatment but do require more intensive treatment than 1 or 2 hours a week of therapy. One form of day treatment, partial hospitalization, arranges care for children who need the treatment offered in a psychiatric hospital during the day but are able to return home in the evening.

Developmental disorders: A set of mental disorders characterized by deviations from the normal path of child development. Such disorders may be pervasive, thereby affecting multiple areas of development (e.g., autism), or specific, affecting only one aspect of development (e.g., arithmetic disorder).

Diagnostic Interview Schedule for Children (DISC): A child-oriented version of the Diagnostic Interview Schedule, a questionnaire developed for use by the National Institute of Mental Health for its epidemiologic catchment area survey of mental disability in adults.

Eating disorders: Psychophysiological disorders characterized by disturbances in eating. Such disorders include anorexia nervosa and bulimia.

Emotional disorders: Mental disorders characterized by the presence of an emotional problem and considerable impairment of a child's ability to function. Such disorders include anxiety and childhood depression.

Encopresis: A psychophysiological disorder characterized by defecation at inappropriate times.

Enuresis: A psychophysiological disorder characterized by involuntary bedwetting or other lack of control over urination.

Family therapy: A type of psychotherapy based on the idea that a child's problems are manifestations of disturbed interactions within a family rather than problems that lie within the child alone. Treatment heavily involves other family members as well as the child (e.g., in sessions attended by the entire family) because it is believed that a child cannot change if the family as a whole does not change.

Group therapy: A type of psychotherapy in which the focus is on helping individuals develop healthier ways of relating to other people, although therapy groups serve other purposes.

Inpatient treatment: Provision of mental health services to persons staying in a hospital overnight.

Integration of services: The establishment of interrelationships among mental health and other service systems (e.g., the educational, health care, welfare, and juvenile justice systems) so that programs to prevent mental health problems can be offered, children in need of mental health services can be identified, and mental health treatment can be provided at the site where problems are identified.

Length of stay (LOS): The number of days between the date of admission to a health care facility and the discharge date.

Mental disorder: In this background paper, any of the diagnoses classified as mental disorders by the American Psychiatric Association in the *Diagnostic and Statistical Manual of Mental Disorders* (DSM-III). Generally, DSM-III defines a mental disorder as a clinically significant behavioral or psychological syndrome or pattern that occurs in an individual and that is typically associated with either a painful symptom (distress) or impairment in one or more areas of functioning (disability).

Mental health problem: In this background paper, either a mental disorder or more general subclinical problem affecting mental health but not meeting the criteria for a diagnosable mental disorder.

Mental health services: Any of the wide range of services designed to meet mental health needs but primarily including therapies and prevention techniques.

Neuroleptics: Any drug (e.g., certain tranquilizers) used to reduce psychotic behavior.

Neurosis: Currently, there is no consensus in the mental health field as to the definition of neurosis, and the category neuroses was not included in DSM-III although it had been included in previous Diagnostic and Statistical Manuals. The term neurosis is usually used to refer to emotional disorders caused by unconscious conflict and characterized chiefly by anxiety.

Outpatient treatment: Provision of mental health services on an ambulatory basis to persons who do not require 24-hour or partial hospitalization. Settings for outpatient treatment include community mental health centers and private mental health practices.

Primary prevention: Efforts to avert mental health

problems altogether. For children, these efforts include interventions directed at parents and educators.

Private psychiatric hospital: A hospital operated privately by individuals, partnerships, corporations, or nonprofit organizations, primarily for the care of persons with serious mental disorders.

Psychodynamic therapy: Psychotherapy based on the theory that changes in cognitions and emotions will be followed by changes in behavior.

Psychopharmacological therapy: Therapy involving the use of psychoactive medications such as stimulants, antidepressants, or neuroleptics.

Psychophysiological disorders: Mental health disorders that involve a disturbance in some aspect of bodily functioning usually involving a combination of mental and physical factors. Such disorders include stereotyped movement disorders; eating disorders such as anorexia and bulimia; and enuresis and encopresis.

Residential treatment center (RTC): A residential facility, not licensed as a psychiatric hospital, whose primary purpose is the provision of individually planned programs of mental health treatment services in conjunction with residential care for children and youths primarily under the age of 18. The term used by NIMH is "residential treatment centers for emotionally disturbed children," but children with other mental disorders are also treated in these facilities.

Secondary prevention: Efforts to detect mental health problems in their early stages of development and to apply techniques to reduce the severity and duration of incipient problems.

State and county mental hospital: A psychiatric hospital that is under the auspices of a State or county government, or operated jointly by both a State and county government.

State Mental Health Agencies (SMHAs): Agencies under the auspices of State governments, staffed through the State, and offering mental health services to State residents in need of mental health care. State mental health agencies may supervise State mental hospitals, CMHCs, RTCs, and/or day treatment facilities.

Stereotyped movement disorders: Psychophysiological disorders characterized by involuntary movements of bodily parts (i.e., tics).

Substance use/abuse disorders: A set of mental disorders characterized by maladaptive behavioral changes resulting from regular use of substances that affect the central nervous system. Substance use and abuse disorders are not classified as childhood-onset mental disorders by DSM-III, but children can be afflicted by them.

Tertiary prevention: Attempts to arrest further deterioration in individuals who already suffer from severe mental health problems (disorders). Treatment can be considered tertiary prevention. The term is not used in this background paper.

References

References

1. Abel, E.L., *Fetal Alcohol Syndrome Volume I: An Annotated and Comprehensive Bibliography* (Boca Raton, FL: CRC Press, 1981).
2. Aber, J.L., "The Socio-Emotional Development of Maltreated Children," unpublished doctoral dissertation, Yale University, New Haven, CT, 1982.
3. Aber, J.L., and Cicchetti, D., "The Socio-Emotional Development of Maltreated Children: An Empirical and Theoretical Analysis," *Theory and Research in Behavioral Pediatrics*, H. Fitzgerald, B. Lester, and M. Yogman (eds.) (New York: Plenum Press, 1984).
4. Abikoff, H., and Gittelman, R., "Does Behavior Therapy Normalize the Classroom Behavior of Hyperactive Children?" *Archives of General Psychiatry* 41:449, 1984.
5. Abramowitz, C.V., "The Effectiveness of Group Psychotherapy With Children," *Archives of General Psychiatry* 33:320, 1976.
6. Abt Associates, *A National Survey of Head Start Graduates and Their Peers*, Contract No. HEW 105-76-1103; ED 152422 (Cambridge, MA: 1978).
7. Achenbach, T.M., "The Classification of Child Psychopathology: A Review and Analysis of Empirical Efforts," *Psychological Bulletin* 85: 1275, 1978.
8. Achenbach, T.M., "Psychopathology of Childhood: Research Problems and Issues," *Journal of Consulting and Clinical Psychology* 46:759, 1978.
9. Achenbach, T.M., *Developmental Psychopathology* (New York: John Wiley & Sons, 1982).
10. Adams, D., *Parent Involvement: Parent Development* (Oakland, CA: Center for the Study of Parent Involvement, 1976).
11. Adams, P.L., "Children and Paraservices of the Community Mental Health Centers," *Journal of the American Academy of Child Psychiatry* 14:18-31, 1975.
12. Adams-Tucker, C., "Proximate Effects of Sexual Abuse in Childhood: A Report on 28 Children," *American Journal of Psychiatry* 139(10): 1252, 1982.
13. Akiskal, H.S., and McKinney, W.T., "Overview of Recent Research in Depression: Integration of Ten Conceptual Models Into a Comprehensive Clinical Frame," *Archives of General Psychiatry* 32:285, 1975.
14. Alabiso, F., "Operant Control of Attention Behavior: A Treatment for Hyperactivity," *Behavior Therapy* 6:39, 1975.
15. Albee, George, "Toward a Just Society: Lessons From Observations on the Primary Prevention of Psychopathology," *American Psychologist* 41(8):891-898, 1986.
16. Alexander, J.F., and Parsons, B.V., "Short-Term Behavioral Intervention With Delinquent Families: Impact on Family Processes and Recidivism," *Journal of Abnormal Psychology* 81:219, 1973.
17. Aman, M.G., "Drugs, Learning and the Psychotherapies," *Pediatric Psychopharmacology: The Use of Behavior Modifying Drugs in Children*, J.S. Werry (ed.) (New York: Brunner/Mazel, 1978).
18. American Humane Association, *Highlights of the 1979 National Data* (Englewood, CO: 1981).
19. American Psychiatric Association, *Diagnostic and Statistical Manual of Mental Disorders*, 3rd ed. (Washington, DC: 1980).
20. American Psychiatric Association, Office of Economic Affairs, "A Review of the Extent of and Trends in Insurance Coverage for Psychiatric Illness in the Private Sector," unpublished, Washington, DC, September 1985.
21. Anderson, D.R., "Prevalence of Behavioral and Emotional Disturbance and Specific Problem Types in a Sample of Disadvantaged Preschool-Aged Children," *Journal of Clinical Child Psychology* 12:130, 1983.
22. Anthony, W., Buell, G., Sharratt, S., et al., "Efficacy of Psychiatric Rehabilitation," *Psychological Bulletin* 78:447, 1972.
23. Appelbaum, A.S., "Developmental Retardation in Infants as a Concomitant of Physical Child Abuse," *Journal of Abnormal Child Psychology* 5:417, 1977.
24. Armstrong, B., "Financing Mental Health Services for Youth: Problems and Possibilities," *Hospital and Community Psychiatry* 29:191, 1978.
25. Armstrong, K.A., "A Treatment and Education Program for Parents and Children Who Are at Risk of Abuse and Neglect," *Child Abuse and Neglect* 5:167, 1981.
26. Armstrong, K.A., "Economic Analysis of a Child Abuse and Neglect Treatment Program," *Child Welfare* 62:3, 1983.
27. Atkeson, B.M., and Forehand, R.L., "Home-Based Reinforcement Programs Designed to Modify Classroom Behavior: A Review and Methodological Evaluation," *Psychological Bulletin* 86(6):1298, 1979.
28. Atkeson, B.M., Forehand, R.L., and Rickard,

K.M., "The Effects of Divorce on Children," *Advances in Clinical Child Psychology*, vol. V, B.B. Lahey and A.E. Kazdin (eds.) (New York: Plenum Press, 1982).

29. Ayllon, T., and Kandel, H.J., "A Behavioral-Educational Alternative to Drug Control of Hyperactive Children," *Journal of Applied Behavioral Analysis* 8:137, 1975.

30. Ayllon, T., and Rosenbaum, M.S., "The Behavioral Treatment of Disruption and Hyperactivity in School Settings," *Advances in Clinical Child Psychology*, vol. I, B.B. Lahey and A.E. Kazdin (eds.) (New York: Plenum Press, 1977).

31. Bachman, J.G., O'Malley, P.M., and Johnston, L.D., "Smoking, Drinking and Drug Use Among American High School Students: Correlates and Trends, 1975-1979," *American Journal of Public Health* 71:59, 1981.

32. Baker, E.L., "Effects of Chronic Illness on Cognitive Development: The Mind, the Body, and the Self," *The Mind of the Child Who Is Said To Be Sick*, D. Copeland, B. Pfefferbaum, and A. Stovall (eds.) (Springfield, IL: Charles C. Thomas, 1983).

33. Bakwin, H., "The Genetics of Bed-Wetting," *Bladder Control and Enuresis*, I. Kolvin, R. MacKeith, and S.R. Meadow (eds.) (London, England: SIMP Heinemann, 1973).

34. Baldwin, J.A., and Oliver, J.E., "Epidemiology and Family Characteristics of Severely Abused Children," *British Journal of Preventive and Social Medicine* 29:205, 1975.

35. Baldwin, W., and Cain, V.S., "The Children of Teenage Parents," *Family Planning Perspectives* 12(1):34, 1980.

36. Balla, D., and Zigler, E., "Mental Retardation," *New Perspectives in Abnormal Psychology*, A.E. Kazdin, A.S. Bellack, and M. Hersen (eds.) (New York: Oxford University Press, 1980).

37. Bandura, A., *Principles of Behavior Modification* (New York: Holt, Rinehart & Winston, 1969).

38. Banta, H.D., and Saxe, L., "Reimbursement for Psychotherapy: Linking Efficacy Research and Public Policy," *American Psychologist* 38:918, 1983.

39. Barahal, R.M., Waterman, J., and Martin, H.P., "The Social Cognitive Development of Abused Children," *Journal of Consulting and Clinical Psychology* 49:508, 1981.

40. Barker, B.L., Heifetz, L.J., and Brightman, A.J., *Parents as Teachers: Manuals for Behavior Modification of the Retarded Child: Studies in Family Training* (Cambridge, MA: Behavioral Educator Projects, 1972).

41. Barkley, R.A., "Learning Disabilities," *Behavioral Assessment of Childhood Disorders*, E. Mash and L. Terdal (eds.) (New York: Guilford Press, 1981).

42. Barkley, R.A., and Cunningham, C.E., "Do Stimulant Drugs Improve the Academic Performance of Hyperactive Children?: A Review of Outcome," *Clinical Pediatrics* 17:85, 1978.

43. Barrett, C.L., Hampe, I.E., and Miller, L.C., "Research on Child Psychotherapy," *Handbook of Psychotherapy and Behavior Change: An Empirical Analysis*, 2nd ed., S. Garfield and A. Bergin (eds.) (New York: John Wiley & Sons, 1978).

44. Beardslee, W.R., Bemporad, J., Keller, M.B., et al., "Children of Parents With Major Affective Disorders: A Review," *American Journal of Psychiatry* 140(7):825, 1983.

45. Bebbington, P.E., "The Epidemiology of Depressive Disorder," *Culture, Medicine and Society*, A.M. Kleinman (ed.) (Dodrecht, The Netherlands: Reidel, 1978).

46. Beckwith, L., and Cohen, S.E., "Interactions of Preterm Infants With Their Caregivers and Test Performance at Age Two," *High Risk Infants and Children: Adult and Peer Interactions*, T.M. Field, S. Goldberg, D. Stern, et al. (eds.) (New York: Academic Press, 1980).

47. Beezley, P., Mrazek, P.B., and Mrazek, D.A., "The Effects of Child Sexual Abuse: Methodological Considerations," *Sexually Abused Children and Their Families*, P.B. Mrazek and C.H. Kempe (eds.) (Oxford, England: Pergamon Press, 1981).

48. Behar, L., "Foster Care: Positive Approaches to a National Problem," *Journal of Clinical Child Psychology* 10(1):2, 1981.

49. Behar, L., "An Integrated System of Services for Seriously Disturbed Children," unpublished paper, National Institute of Justice/Alcohol, Drug Abuse and Mental Health Administration Conference, Washington, DC, 1984.

50. Behar, L., "Changing Patterns of State Responsibility: A Case Study of North Carolina," *Journal of Clinical Child Psychology* 14:188, 1985.

51. Bell, R.W., and Smotherman, W.P. (eds.), *Maternal Injuries and Early Behavior* (New York: Spectrum Publications, 1980).

52. Belmont, L., and Dryfoos, J., "Long-Term Development of Children Born to New York City Teenagers," *Teenage Parents and Their Offspring*, K.G. Scott, T. Field, and E. Robertson (eds.) (New York: Grune & Stratton, 1981).

53. Belsky, J., "Testimony Before the U.S. House of Representatives, September 5, 1984, on the Sub-

ject of Infant Day Care and Child Development," American Psychological Association, Washington, DC, 1984.

54. Bemis, K.M., "Current Approaches to the Etiology and Treatment of Anorexia Nervosa," *Psychological Bulletin* 85:593, 1978.

55. Berlin, I.N., "Some Models for Reversing the Myth of Child Treatment in Community Mental Health Centers," *Journal of the American Academy of Child Psychiatry* 14:76, 1975.

56. Berreuter-Clement, J., Schweinhart, L., Barnett, W., et al., *Changed Lives: The Effects of the Perry Preschool Program on Youths Through Age 19* (Ypsilanti, MI: High/Scope Educational Research Foundation, 1984).

57. Besharov, D.J., "U.S. National Center on Child Abuse and Neglect: Three Years of Experience," *International Journal of Child Abuse and Neglect* 1:173, 1977.

58. Bettelheim, B., *The Empty Fortress* (New York: Free Press, 1967).

59. Black, C., "Children of Alcoholics," *Alcohol Health and Research World* 4:23, 1979.

60. Blinder, B.J., Young, W.M., Fineman, K.R., et al., "The Children's Psychiatric Unit in the Community: Concept and Development," *American Journal of Psychiatry* 135(7):848, 1978.

61. Blotcky, M.J., Dimperio, T.L., and Gossett, J.T., "Followup of Children Treated in Psychiatric Hospitals: A Review of Studies," *American Journal of Psychiatry* 141(12):1499, 1984.

62. Blouin, A.G.A., Bornstein, R.A., and Trites, R.L., "Teenage Alcohol Abuse Among Hyperactive Children: A Five-Year Follow-Up Study," *Journal of Pediatric Psychology* 3:188, 1978.

63. Blum, A., and Singer, M., "Substance Abuse and Social Deviance: A Youth Assessment Framework," *Adolescent Substance Abuse: A Guide to Prevention and Treatment*, R. Israelowitz and M. Singer (eds.) (New York: Haworth Press, 1983).

64. Boskind-Lodahl, M., and White, W.C., "The Definition and Treatment of Bulimarexia in College Women—A Pilot Study," *Journal of the American College Health Association* 27:84, 1978.

65. Boszormenyi-Nagy, I., and Ulrich, D.N., "Contextual Family Therapy," *Handbook of Family Therapy*, A.S. Gurman and D.P. Kniskern (eds.) (New York: Brunner/Mazel, 1981).

66. Bousha, D., and Twentyman, C, "Abusing, Neglectful, and Comparison Mother-Child Interactional Style: Naturalistic Observations in the Home Setting," *Journal of Abnormal Psychology*, in press.

67. Bowen, M., "Family Therapy and Family Group Therapy," *Treating Relationships*, D. Olson (ed.) (Lake Mills, IA: Graphic Publishing, 1975).

68. Boyar, R.M., Katz, J., Finkelstein, J.W., et al., "Anorexia Nervosa: Immaturity of the 24-hour Luteinizing Hormone Secretory Pattern," *New England Journal of Medicine* 291:861, 1974.

69. Boyd, J.H., and Weissman, M.M., "Epidemiology of Affective Disorders: A Reexamination and Future Directions," *Archives of General Psychiatry* 38:1039, 1981.

70. Boyd, J.H., and Weissman, M.M., "Epidemiology," *Handbook of Affective Disorders*, E.S. Paykel (ed.) (New York: Guilford Press, 1982).

71. Boyle, I.R., deSanté Agnese, P.A., Sack, S., et al., "Emotional Adjustment of Adolescents and Young Adults With Cystic Fibrosis," *Journal of Pediatrics* 88:313, 1976.

72. Bradley, K.H., Balow, E.A., and Bruininks, R.H., "A National Study of Prescribed Drugs in Institutions and Community Residential Facilities for Mentally Retarded People," *Psychopharmacology Bulletin* 279, 1985.

73. Bremburg, S., "Pregnancy in Swedish Teenagers: Perinatal Problems and Social Situation," *Scandinavian Journal of Social Medicine* 5(1):15, 1977.

74. Breslau, N., "Psychiatric Disorder in Children With Physical Disabilities," *Journal of the American Academy of Child Psychiatry* 24(1):87, 1985.

75. Breuning, S.E., and Davidson, N.A., "Effects of Psychotropic Drugs on Intelligence Test Performance of Institutionalized Mentally Retarded Adults," *American Journal of Mental Deficiency* 85:575, 1981.

76. Broman, S.H., "Long-Term Development of Children Born to Teenagers," *Teenage Parents and Their Offspring*, K.G. Scott, T. Field, and E.G. Robertson (eds.) (New York: Grune & Stratton, 1981).

77. Bronfenbrenner, U., "Is Early Intervention Effective?" *Handbook of Evaluation Research*, M. Guttentag and E.L. Struening (eds.) (Beverly Hills, CA: Sage, 1975).

78. Broussard, E.R., "Evaluation of Televised Anticipatory Guidance to Primiparae," *Community Mental Health Journal* 12:203, 1976.

79. Brown, B.S., "Foreword," *Dyslexia: An Appraisal of Current Knowledge*, A. Benton and D. Pear (eds.) (New York: Oxford University Press, 1978).

80. Brown, J.V., and Bakeman, R., "Relationships of Human Mothers With Their Infants During the First Year of Life: Effect of Prematurity,"

Maternal Injuries and Early Behavior, R.W. Bell and W.P. Smotherman (eds.) (New York: Spectrum Publications, 1980).

81. Brown, R.T., Broden, K.A., and Clingerman, S.R., "Pharmacotherapy in ADD Adolescents With Special Attention to Multimodality Treatments," *Psychopharmacology Bulletin* 21(2):192, 1985.

82. Bryan, T., "Peer Popularity of Learning Disabled Children: A Replication," *Journal of Learning Disabilities* 9:49, 1976.

83. Bryant, B., "Special Foster Care: A History and Rationale," *Journal of Clinical Child Psychology* 10:8, 1981.

84. Buchanan, A., and Oliver, J.E., "Abuse and Neglect as a Cause of Mental Retardation: A Study of 140 Children Admitted to Subnormality Hospitals in Wiltshire," *British Journal of Psychiatry* 131:458, 1977.

85. Burns, B.J., and Cromer, W.W., "The Evolving Role of the Psychologist in Primary Health Care Practitioner Training for Mental Health Science," *Journal of Clinical Child Psychology* 4(1):8, 1978.

86. Buzogany, W., "So You Want To Start a Juvenile Justice/Mental Health Inpatient Unit?" *Addressing the Mental Health Needs of the Juvenile Justice Population: Policies and Programs*, symposium cosponsored by the National Association of State Mental Health Program Directors and the National Institute of Mental Health held in conjunction with the winter meeting of the State Mental Health Representatives for Children and Youth, Washington, DC, Feb. 27-28, 1985.

87. Cadonet, R.J., "Psychopathology in Adopted-Away Offspring of Biological Parents With Antisocial Behavior," *Archives of General Psychiatry* 35:176, 1978.

88. Camp, B.W., Blom, G.E., Herbert, F., et al., " 'Think Aloud': A Program for Developing Self-Control in Young Aggressive Boys," *Journal of Abnormal Child Psychology* 5:157, 1977.

89. Campbell, M., "Schizophrenic Disorders and Pervasive Developmental Disorders/Infantile Autism," *Diagnosis and Psychopharmacology of Childhood and Adolescent Disorders*, J. Wiener (ed.) (New York: John Wiley & Sons, 1985).

90. Campbell, M., Anderson, L.T., Meier, M., et al., "A Comparison of Haloperidol and Behavior Therapy and Their Interaction in Autistic Children," *Journal of the American Academy of Child Psychiatry* 17:640, 1978.

91. Campbell, M., Anderson, L.T., Small, A.M., et al., "The Effects of Haloperidol on Learning and Behavior in Autistic Children," *Journal of Autism and Developmental Disorders* 12:167, 1982.

92. Campbell, M., Green, W.H., Perry, R., et al., "Pharmacotherapy," *Handbook of Clinical Child Psychology*, C.E. Walker and M.C. Roberts (eds.) (New York: John Wiley & Sons, 1983).

93. Cantor, P., "Depression and Suicide in Children," *Handbook of Clinical Child Psychology*, C. Walker and M. Roberts (eds.) (New York: John Wiley & Sons, 1983).

94. Cantwell, D.P., "Childhood Depression: A Review of Current Research," *Advances in Clinical Child Psychology*, B.B. Lahey and A.E. Kazdin (eds.) (New York: Plenum Press, 1982).

95. Cantwell, D.P., "Childhood Depression: What Do We Know, Where Do We Go?" *Childhood Psychopathology and Development*, S.B. Guze, F.J. Earls, and J.E. Barrett (eds.) (New York: Raven Press, 1983).

96. Cantwell, D.P., and Carlson, G.A., "Stimulants," *Pediatric Psychopharmacology: The Use of Behavior Modifying Drugs in Children*, J.S. Werry (ed.) (New York: Brunner/Mazel, 1978).

97. Cantwell, D.P., Baker, L., and Rutter, M., "Families of Autistic and Dysphasic Children," *Archives of General Psychiatry* 36:682, 1979.

98. Caplan, G., *Principles of Preventive Psychiatry* (New York: Basic Books, 1964).

99. Caputo, D.V., and Mandell, W., "Consequences of Low Birth Weight," *Developmental Psychology* 3:363, 1970.

100. Caputo, D.V., Goldstein, K.M., and Taub, H.B., "The Development of Prematurely Born Children Through Middle Childhood," *Infants Born at Risk*, T.M. Field, A.M. Sostek, S. Goldberg, et al. (eds.) (New York: Spectrum Publications, 1979).

101. Card, J.J., *Long-Term Consequences for Children Born to Adolescent Parents*, final report to the National Institute of Child Health and Human Development, National Institutes of Health, Public Health Service, U.S. Department of Health and Human Services (Washington, DC: U.S. Government Printing Office, 1978).

102. Carlson, G.A., and Cantwell, D.P., "Unmasking Masked Depression in Children and Adolescents," *American Journal of Psychiatry* 137(4): 445, 1980.

103. Carlson, G.A., and Cantwell, D.P., "Suicidal Behavior and Depression in Children and Adolescents," *Journal of the American Academy of Child Psychiatry* 21:361, 1982.

104. Casey, R.J., and Berman, J.S., "The Outcome

of Psychotherapy With Children," *Psychological Bulletin* 98:388, 1985.

105. Casper, R.C., Eckert, E.D., Halmi, K.A., et al., "Bulimia: Its Incidence and Clinical Importance in Patients With Anorexia Nervosa," *Archives of General Psychiatry* 37:1030, 1980.

106. Cass, L.K., and Thomas, C.B., *Childhood Pathology and Later Adjustment* (New York: John Wiley & Sons, 1979).

107. Chandler, C.L., Weissberg, R.P, Cowen, E.L., et al., "Long-Term Effects of a School-Based Secondary Prevention Program for Young Maladapting Children," *Journal of Consulting and Clinical Psychology* 52:165, 1984.

108. Children's Defense Fund, *Children Without Homes* (Washington, DC: 1978).

109. Children's Defense Fund, *A Children's Defense Budget* (Washington, DC: 1985).

110. Chilman, C.S., "Programs for Disadvantaged Parents: Some Major Trends and Related Research," *Review of Child Development Research*, B.M. Caldwell and H.N. Ricciute (eds.) (Chicago, IL: University of Chicago Press, 1973).

111. Chilman, C.S., *Adolescent Sexuality in a Changing American Society* (New York: John Wiley & Sons, 1983).

112. Christophersen, E.R., and Rapoff, M.A., "Pediatric Psychology: An Appraisal," *Advances in Clinical Child Psychology*, vol. 3, B.B. Lahey and A.E. Kazdin (eds.) (New York: Plenum Press, 1980).

113. Cicirelli, V.G., *The Impact of Head Start: An Evaluation of the Effects of Head Start on Children's Cognitive and Affective Development* (Washington, DC: National Bureau of Standards, Institute for Applied Technology, 1969).

114. Cleland, C.C., "Mental Retardation," *Handbook of Clinical Child Psychology*, C. Walker and M. Roberts (eds.) (New York: John Wiley & Sons, 1983).

115. Cohler, B.J., Grunebaum, H.U., Weiss, J.L., et al., "Disturbance of Attention Among Schizophrenic, Depressed and Well Mothers and Their Children," *Journal of Child Psychology and Psychiatry* 18:115, 1977.

116. Comer, J., "The Yale-New Haven Primary Prevention Project: A Follow-up Study," *Journal of the American Academy of Child Psychiatry* 24:154, 1985.

117. Comer, J., and Hill, H., "Social Policy and the Mental Health of Black Children," *Journal of the American Academy of Child Psychiatry* 24:175-181, 1985.

118. Comer, J.P., and Schraft, C.M., "Working With Black Parents," *Parent Education and Intervention Handbook*, R.R. Abidin (ed.) (Springfield, IL: Charles C. Thomas, 1980).

119. Committee on Child Psychiatry, *From Diagnosis to Treatment; An Approach to Treatment Planning for the Emotionally Disturbed Child*, vol. 8, Report No. 87 (New York: Group for the Advancement of Psychiatry, 1973).

120. "Complex Problems of Teen-Age Pregnancy," *New York Times*, p. 48, Mar. 2, 1985.

121. Conners, C.K., and Werry, J.S., "Pharmacotherapy," *Psychopathological Disorders of Childhood*, H.C. Quay and J.S. Werry (eds.) (New York: John Wiley & Sons, 1979).

122. Conte, J.R., and Berliner, L., "Sexual Abuse of Children: Implications for Practice," *Social Casework* 62:601, 1981.

123. Cooper, T., "Present HEW Policies in Primary Prevention," *Preventive Medicine* 6(2):198, 1977.

124. Corrigan, F.C., Berger, S.J., Dienstbier, R.A., et al., "The Influence of Prematurity on School Performance," *American Journal of Mental Deficiency* 71:533, 1967.

125. Cowen, E.L., Davidson, E., and Gesten, E.L., "Program Dissemination and the Modification of Delivery Practices in School Mental Health," *Professional Psychology* 11:36, 1980.

126. Cowen, E.L., Gesten, E.L., and Weissberg, R.P., "An Interrelated Network of Preventively Oriented School Based Mental Health Approaches," *Evaluation and Action in the Community Context*, R.H. Price and P. Politzer (eds.) (New York: Academic Press, 1980).

127. Cowen, E.L., Pederson, A., Babigian, H., et al., "Long-Term Follow-Up of Early Detected Vulnerable Children," *Journal of Consulting and Clinical Psychology* 41:438, 1973.

128. Cowen, E.L., Trost, M.A., Lorion, R.P., et al., *New Ways in School Mental Health: Early Detection and Prevention of School Maladaption* (New York: Human Science Press, 1975).

129. Craighead, W.E., Wilcoxon-Craighead, L., and Meyers, A.W., "New Directions in Behavior Modification With Children," *Progress in Behavior Modification*, vol. 4, M. Hersen, R.M. Eisler, and P.M. Miller (eds.) (New York: Academic Press, 1978).

130. Crnic, K.A., Greenberg, M.T., Ragozin, A.S., et al., "Effects of Stress and Social Support on Mothers and Premature and Full-Term Infants," *Child Development* 54:129, 1983.

131. Crook, T., and Raskin, A., "Association of

Childhood Parental Love With Attempted Suicide and Depression," *Journal of Consulting and Clinical Psychology* 43:277, 1975.

132. Cunningham, C.E., and Barkley, R.A., "The Role of Academic Failure in Hyperactive Behavior," *Journal of Learning Disabilities* 11:15, 1978.

133. Cytryn, L., and McKnew, D.H., "Factors Influencing the Changing Clinical Expression of the Depressive Process in Children," *American Journal of Psychiatry* 131:879, 1974.

134. Datta, L., "The Impact of the Westinghouse-Ohio Evaluation of the Development of the Project Head Start: An Examination of the Immediate and Longer-Term Effects and How They Came About," *The Evaluation of Social Programs*, C.C. Abt (ed.) (Beverly Hills, CA: Sage, 1976).

135. Davenport, Y.B., Zahn-Waxler, C., Adland, M.L., et al., "Early Child-Rearing Practices in Families With a Manic-Depressive Parent," *American Journal of Psychiatry* 141(2):230, 1984.

136. Davidson, W.S., and Seidman, E., "Studies of Behavior Modification and Juvenile Delinquency: A Review, Methodological Critique and Social Perspective," *Psychological Bulletin* 81:998, 1974.

137. Davie, R., Butler, N., and Goldstein, H., *From Birth to Seven: A Report of the National Child Development Study* (London, England: Longman Group, Ltd., 1972).

138. Davies, P., "Outlook for Low Birthweight Children—Then and Now," *Archives of Diseases in Childhood* 51:817, 1976.

139. Day, J.R., "Treatment Models for Adolescents: Residential Treatment Centers Versus Hospitals," *Journal of the National Association of Private Psychiatric Hospitals* 4(4):1972-1973.

140. DeHirsh, K., Jansky, J., and Langford, W.S., "Comparisons Between Prematurely and Maturely Born Children at Three Age Levels," *American Journal of Orthopsychiatry* 36:616, 1966.

141. DeLeon, P.H., and VandenBos, G.R., "Psychotherapy Reimbursement in Federal Programs," *Psychotherapy: Practice, Research and Policy*, G.R. VandenBos (ed.) (Beverly Hills, CA: Sage, 1980).

142. DeLissovoy, V., "Child Care by Adolescent Parents," *Children Today* 2:22, 1975.

143. Denney, D.R., "Reflection and Impulsivity as Determinants of Conceptual Strategy," *Child Development* 44:614, 1973.

144. Deutsch, C.P., "Social Class and Child Development," *Review of Child Development Research*, vol. 3, B.M. Caldwell and H.R. Ricciuti (eds.) (Chicago, IL: University of Chicago Press, 1973).

145. DeVitto, B., and Goldberg, S., "The Effects of Newborn Medical Status on Early Parent-Infant Interaction," *Infants Born at Risk*, T.M. Field, A.M. Sostek, S. Goldberg, et al. (eds.) (New York: Spectrum Publications, 1979).

146. Dietrich, K.N., Starr, R.H., and Kaplan, M.G., "Maternal Stimulation and Care of Abused Infants," *High Risk Infants and Children*, T.M. Field, S. Goldberg, D. Stern, et al. (eds.) (New York: Academic Press, 1980).

147. Doleys, D.M., "Assessment and Treatment of Enuresis and Encopresis in Children," *Progress in Behavior Modification*, vol. 4, M. Hersen, R.M. Eisler, and P.M. Miller (eds.) (New York: Academic Press, 1978).

148. Douglas, J., and Gear, R., "Children of Low Birth Weight in the 1946 Cohort," *Archives of Diseases of Children* 51:820, 1976.

149. Dreger, R.M., and Miller, K.S., "Comparative Psychological Studies of Negroes and Whites in the United States," *Psychological Bulletin* 57:361, 1960.

150. Dreger, R.M., and Miller, K.S., "Comparative Psychological Studies of Negroes and Whites in the United States: 1959-1965," *Psychological Bulletin* 70:1, 1968.

151. Drotar, D., "Adaptational Problems of Children and Adolescents With Cystic Fibrosis," *Journal of Pediatric Psychology* 3:45, 1978.

152. Drotar, D., "Psychological Perspectives in Chronic Childhood Illness," *Journal of Pediatric Psychology* 6(3):211, 1981.

153. Drotar, D., "Research and Practice in Failure to Thrive: The State of the Art," *Zero to Three* 5(3):1, 1985.

154. Drotar, D., Crawford, P., and Bush, M., "The Family Context of Childhood Chronic Illness: Implications for Psychosocial Intervention," *Chronic Illness and Disability Through the Life Span Effects on Self and Family*, vol. 4, M.G. Eisenberg, L.C. Sutkin, and M.A. Ansen (eds.) (New York: Springer, 1984).

155. Drotar, D., Doershuk, C.F., Stern, R.C., et al., "Psychosocial Functioning of Children With Cystic Fibrosis," *Pediatrics* 67:338, 1981.

156. Duncan, F.D., "Life Stress as a Precursor to Adolescent Drug Dependence," *International Journal of Addiction* 12:1047, 1977.

157. Durlak, J.A., "Providing Mental Health Services to Elementary School Children," *Handbook of*

Clinical Child Psychology, C. Walker and M. Roberts (eds.) (New York: John Wiley & Sons, 1983).

158. Durlak, J.A., and Jason, L.A., "Preventive Programs for School-Aged Children and Adolescents," *Prevention of Problems in Childhood*, M.C. Roberts and L. Peterson (eds.) (New York: John Wiley & Sons, 1984).

159. Ebbin, A.J., Gollub, M.H., Stein, A.M., et al., "Battered Child Syndrome at the Los Angeles County General Hospital," *American Journal of Diseases of Children* 118:660, 1969.

160. Edelbrook, C., "Running Away From Home: Incidence and Correlates Among Children and Youth Referred for Mental Health Services," *Journal of Family Issues* 1:210, 1980.

161. Egan, J., testimony in *Emerging Trends in Mental Health Care for Adolescents*, Hearing Before the Select Committee on Children, Youth and Families, House of Representatives, U.S. Congress, Washington, DC, June 6, 1985.

162. Egeland, B., and Sroufe, L.A., "Developmental Sequelae of Maltreatment in Infancy," *New Directions for Child Development: Developmental Perspectives on Child Maltreatment*, No. 11, R. Rizley, and D. Cicchetti (eds.) (San Francisco, CA: Jossey-Bass, Inc., 1981).

163. Egeland, B., Sroufe, L.A., and Erickson, M., "The Development Consequences of Different Patterns of Maltreatment," *Child Abuse and Neglect* 7:459, 1983.

164. Egeland, B., Wozniak, R., Schrimpf, V., et al., "Visual Information Processing: Evaluation of a Training Program for Children With Learning Disabilities," paper presented at the American Educational Research Association Convention, San Francisco, CA, April 1976.

165. El-Guebaly, N., and Offord, D.R., "The Offspring of Alcoholics: A Critical Review," *American Journal of Psychiatry* 134(4):357, 1977.

166. El-Guebaly, N., and Offord, D.R., "On Being the Offspring of an Alcoholic: An Update," *Alcoholism: Clinical and Experimental Research* 3(2):148, 1979.

167. Elmer, E., *Fragile Families, Troubled Children* (Pittsburgh, PA: University of Pittsburgh Press, 1977).

168. Elmer, E., and Gregg, G.S., "Developmental Characteristics of Abused Children," *Pediatrics* 40:596, 1967.

169. Emery, R.E., "Interparental Conflict and the Children of Discord and Divorce," *Psychological Bulletin* 92:310, 1982.

170. Emery, R.E., and Marholin, D., "An Applied Behavior Analysis of Delinquency: The Irrelevancy of Relevant Behavior," *American Psychologist* 32:860, 1977.

171. Erickson, M.N., "Indirect Hypnotic Therapy of a Bedwetting Couple," *Journal of Clinical and Experimental Hypnosis* 2:171, 1954.

172. Erickson, M.N., and Rossi, E.L., *Hypnotic Therapy: An Exploratory Casebook* (New York: Irvingston, 1979).

173. Erickson, R., "Outcome Studies in Mental Hospitals: A Review," *Psychological Bulletin* 82:519, 1975.

174. Eysenck, H.J., "An Exercise in Megasilliness," *American Psychologist* 33:517, 1978.

175. Fagan, J.A., "Residential Treatment for Mentally Disordered Juvenile Offenders," *Addressing the Mental Health Needs of the Juvenile Justice Population: Policies and Programs*, symposium cosponsored by the National Association of State Mental Health Program Directors and the National Institute of Mental Health held in conjunction with the winter meeting of the State Mental Health Representatives for Children and Youth, Washington, DC, Feb. 27-28, 1985.

176. Feingold, B.F., *Why Your Child Is Hyperactive* (New York: Random House, 1975).

177. Fetter, R.B., Shin, Y., Freema, J.L., et al., "Case Mix Definition by Diagnostic Related Groups," *Medical Care* 18:1, 1980.

178. Feuerberg, M., "Provider Types, Settings, Utilization and Expenditures for Mental Health Conditions," paper presented at Annual Convention of the American Psychological Association, Toronto, Ontario, August 1984.

179. Field, T.M., "Effects of Early Separation, Interactive Defects, and Experimental Manipulations on Infant-Mother Face-to-Face Interaction," *Child Development* 48:763, 1977.

180. Field, T.M., "Maternal Stimulation During Infant Feeding," *Developmental Psychology* 13:539, 1977.

181. Field, T.M., "Interaction Patterns of Preterm and Term Infants," *Infants Born at Risk*, T.M. Field, A.M. Sostek, S. Goldberg, et al. (eds.) (New York: Spectrum Publications, 1979).

182. Field, T.M. (ed.), *High Risk Infants and Children: Adult and Peer Interactions* (New York: Academic Press, 1980).

183. Field, T.M., "Early Development of the Preterm Offspring," *Teenage Parents and Their Offspring*, K.G. Scott, T. Field, and E. Robertson (eds.) (New York: Grune & Stratton, 1981).

184. Field, T.M., Dempsey, J., and Shuman, H.H., "Developmental Assessments of Infants Surviving the Respiratory Distress Syndrome," *Infants Born at Risk*, T.M. Field, A.M. Sostek, S. Gold-

berg, et al. (eds.) (New York: Spectrum Publications, 1979).

185. Field, T.M., Dempsey, J., and Shuman, H.H., "Developmental Follow-Up of Pre- and Post-Term Infants," *Preterm Birth and Psychological Development*, S.L. Friedman and M. Sigman (eds.) (New York: Academic Press, 1981).

186. Field, T.M., Dempsey, J., and Shuman, H.H., "Five-Year Follow-Up of Preterm Respiratory Distress Syndrome and Post-Term Postmaturity Syndrome Infants," *Infants Born at Risk*, T. Field and A.M. Sostek (eds.) (New York: Grune & Stratton, 1983).

187. Field, T.M., Widmayer, S.M., Stringer, S., et al., "Teenage, Lower-Class Black Mothers and Their Preterm Infants: An Intervention and Developmental Follow-Up," *Child Development* 51:426, 1980.

188. Fielding, J.E., "Adolescent Pregnancy Revisited," *New England Journal of Medicine* 299(16):893, 1978.

189. Finch, S.M., and Poznanski, E.O., *Adolescent Suicide* (Springfield, IL: Charles C. Thomas, 1971).

190. Finkelhor, D., *Sexually Victimized Children* (New York: Free Press, 1979).

191. Finkelhor, D., "Sexual Abuse: A Sociological Perspective," *Child Abuse and Neglect* 6(1):95, 1982.

192. Fisher, L., and Jones, J.E., "Child Competence and Psychiatric Risk, II: Areas of Relationship Between Child and Family Functioning," *Journal of Nervous and Mental Diseases* 168:332, 1980.

193. Fishman, M., "A Growing Concern: Adolescent Suicide," *Eleventh Annual Report on the Child and Youth Activities* (Washington, DC: National Institute of Mental Health, Alcohol, Drug Abuse, and Mental Health Administration, Public Health Service, U.S. Department of Health and Human Services, 1984).

194. Fitch, M.J., Cadol, R.V., Goldson, E., et al., "Cognitive Development of Abused and Failure-To-Thrive Children," *Journal of Pediatric Psychology* 1:32, 1976.

195. Fitzhardinge, P.M., Pape, K., Artikaitis, M., et al., "Mechanical Ventilation of Infants of Less Than 1500 gm. Birth Weight: Health, Growth, and Neurologic Sequelae," *Journal of Pediatrics* 88:531, 1976.

196. Fleischman, M.J., "A Replication of Patterson's 'Intervention for Boys With Conduct Problems'," *Journal of Consulting and Clinical Psychology* 49:343, 1981.

197. Fleischman, M.J., and Szykula, S.A., "A Community Setting Replication of a Social Learning Treatment for Aggressive Children," *Behavior Therapy* 12:115, 1981.

198. Fogel, R.L., "Early Observations on States' Plans To Provide Children's Mental Health Services Under the ADAMH Block Grant (GAO/HRD-85-84)," letter to Senator Inouye from Human Resources Division, General Accounting Office, U.S. Congress, Washington, DC, July 10, 1985.

199. Fomufod, A., Sinkford, S., and Lovy, V., "Mother-Child Separation at Birth: A Contributing Factor in Child Abuse," *Lancet* 2:549, 1975.

200. Ford, K., "Second Pregnancies Among Teenage Mothers," *Family Planning Perspectives* 15(6):268, 1983.

201. Forehand, R.L., Walley, P.B., and Furey, W.M., "Prevention in the Home: Parent and Family," *Prevention of Problems in Childhood*, M.C. Roberts and L. Peterson (eds.) (New York: John Wiley & Sons, 1984).

202. Fraley, Y.L., "The Family Support Center: Early Intervention for High-Risk Parents and Children," *Children Today* 12(1):13, January to February 1983.

203. Framo, J.L., "Family Theory and Therapy," *American Psychologist* 34(10):988, 1979.

204. Frances-Williams, J., and Davies, P.A., "Very Low Birthweight and Later Intelligence," *Developmental Medicine and Child Neurology* 16:709, 1974.

205. Frank, G., "Treatment Needs of Children in Foster Care," *American Journal of Orthopsychiatry* 50(2):256, 1980.

206. Frank, R.G., and McGuire, T.G., "A Review of Studies of the Impact of Insurance on the Demand and Utilization of Specialty Mental Health Services," *Health Services Research* 21(2):241-265, June 1986.

207. Freedheim, D.K., and Russ, S.R., "Psychotherapy With Children," *Handbook of Clinical Child Psychology*, C.E. Walker and M.C. Roberts (eds.) (New York: John Wiley & Sons, 1983).

208. Friedman, R.M., and Quick, J., "Day Treatment for Adolescents: A Five-Year Status Report," Department of Technical Assistance and Consultation, Florida Mental Health Institute, University of South Florida, Tampa, FL, June 1983.

209. Friedman, R.M., and Street, S., "Admission and Discharge Criteria for Children's Mental Health Services: A Review of the Issues," paper presented at the Department of Epidemiology and Policy Analysis, Florida Mental Health Institute, University of South Florida, Tampa, FL, July 1984.

210. Friedman, S.L., and Sigman, M., *Preterm Birth*

and Psychological Development (New York: Academic Press, 1981).

211. Friedrich, W.N., and Einbender, A.J., "The Abused Child: A Psychological Review," *Journal of Clinical Child Psychology* 12:244, 1983.

212. Friedrich, W.N., Einbender, A.J., and Luecke, W.J., "Cognitive and Behavioral Characteristics of Physically Abused Children," *Journal of Consulting and Clinical Psychology* 51:313, 1983.

213. Furstenberg, F.F., *Unplanned Parenthood* (New York: Free Press, 1976).

214. Gaensbauer, T.J., and Sands, K., "Distorted Affective Communication in Abused/Neglected Infants and Their Potential Impact on Caretakers," *Journal of the American Academy of Child Psychiatry* 18:236, 1979.

215. Gaensbauer, T.J., Harmon, R.J., Lytryn, L., et al., "Social and Affective Development in Infants With a Manic-Depressive Parent," *American Journal of Psychiatry* 141(2):223, 1984.

216. Gair, D.S., "What Systems of Service Delivery Are Needed," unpublished paper, presented at the National Conference on Chronic Mental Illness in Children and Adolescents, Dallas, TX, 1985.

217. Galdston, R., "Observations on Children Who Have Been Physically Abused and Their Parents," *American Journal of Psychiatry* 122:440, 1965.

218. Gamer, E., Gallant, D., Grunebaum, H.U., "Children of Psychotic Mothers: Performance of Three-Year-Old Children on Tests of Attention," *Archives of General Psychiatry* 34:592, 1977.

219. Garbarino, J., "A Preliminary Study of Some Ecological Correlates of Child Abuse: The Impact of Socioeconomic Stress on Mothers," *Child Development* 47:178, 1976.

220. Gardos, G., Cole, J.O., and Tarsy, D., "Withdrawal Syndromes Associated With Antipsychotic Drugs," *American Journal of Psychiatry* 135:1321, 1978.

221. Garmezy, N., and Devine, V., "Project Competence: The Minnesota Studies of Children Vulnerable to Psychopathology," *Children at Risk for Schizophrenia: A Longitudinal Perspective*, N.F. Watt, E.J. Anthony, L.C. Wynne, et al. (eds.) (Cambridge, England: Cambridge University Press, 1984).

222. Gelles, R.J., and Strauss, M.A., "Violence in the American Family," *Journal of Social Issues* 35:15, 1979.

223. George, C., and Main, M., "Social Interactions of Young Abused Children: Approach, Avoidance, and Aggression," *Child Development* 50:306, 1979.

224. George, C., and Main, M., "Abused Children: Their Rejection of Peers and Caregivers," *High Risk Infants and Children: Adult and Peer Interactions*, T.M. Field, S. Goldberg, and D. Stern (eds.) (New York: Academic Press, 1980).

225. Gershon, B., Dunner, D., and Goodwin, R., "Toward a Biology of Affective Disorders," *Archives of General Psychiatry* 25:1, 1971.

226. Gettinger, M., "Treating Behavior Disorders in the Classroom Setting: Recent Advances," presented at the American Psychological Association Convention in Toronto, Ontario, 1984.

227. Gibbens, T.C.N., and Prince, J., *Child Victims of Sex Offences* (London, England: Institute for the Study and Treatment of Delinquency, 1963).

228. Gil, D.G., *Violence Against Children: Physical Abuse in the United States* (Cambridge, MA: Harvard University Press, 1970).

229. Gilmore, L.M., Chang, C., and Coron, D., "Defining and Counting Mentally Ill Children and Adolescents," *A Technical Assistance Package for the Child and Adolescence Service System Program*, vol. II (Rockville, MD: National Institute of Mental Health, Alcohol, Drug Abuse, and Mental Health Administration, Public Health Service, U.S. Department of Health and Human Services, July 1984).

230. Ginott, H., *Group Psychotherapy With Children* (New York: MacMillan, 1961).

231. Giovannoni, J.M., and Becerra, R.M., *Defining Child Abuse* (New York: Free Press, 1979).

232. Gittleman-Klein, R., "Pharmacotherapy and Management of Pathological Separation Anxiety," *Recent Advances in Child Psychopharmacology*, R. Gittleman-Klein (ed.) (New York: Human Science Press, 1975).

233. Gittleman-Klein, R., and Klein, D.F., "Controlled Imipramine Treatment of School Phobia," *Archives of General Psychiatry* 25:204, 1971.

234. Gittleman-Klein, R., Spitzer, R.L., and Cantwell, D., "Diagnostic Classifications and Psychopharmacological Indications," *Pediatric Psychopharmacology*, V.S. Werry (ed.) (New York: Brunner/Mazel, 1978).

235. Glasgow, R.E., and Rosen, G.M., "Behavioral Bibliography: A Review of Self-Help Behavior Manuals," *Psychological Bulletin* 85:1, 1978.

236. Glick, P.C., "Children of Divorced Parents in Demographic Perspective," *Journal of Social Issues* 35:170, 1979.

237. Gogan, J., Koocher, G.P., Fine W.E., et al., "Pediatric Cancer Survival and Marriage: Issues Affecting Adult Adjustment," *American Journal of Orthopsychiatry* 49:423, 1979.

238. Goldberg, E.R., "Depression and Suicide Idea-

tion in the Young Adult," *American Journal of Psychiatry* 138:35, 1981.

239. Goldberg, F., Roghmann, K.J., McInerney, T.K., et al., "Mental Health Problems Among Children Seen in Pediatric Practice," *Pediatrics* 73(3):278-93, 1984.

240. Goldberg, I.D., Regier, D.A., McInerny, T.K., et al., "The Role of the Pediatrician in the Delivery of Mental Health Services to Children," *Pediatrics* 63(6):898, 1979.

241. Golden, M., and Birns, B., "Social Class and Infant Intelligence," *Origins of Intelligence: Infancy and Early Childhood*, M. Lewis (ed.) (New York: Plenum Press, 1976).

242. Gordon, T., *Parent Effectiveness Training: The Tested New Way To Raise Responsible Children* (New York: Wyden, 1970).

243. Gordon, T., and Sands, J.G., *P.E.T. in Action* (New York: Wyden, 1976).

244. Gornick, M., Greenberg, J.N., Eggers, P.W., et al., "Twenty Years of Medicare and Medicaid: Covered Populations, Use of Benefits, and Program Expenditures," *Health Care Financing Review, 1985 Annual Supplement* (Baltimore, MD: Health Care Financing Administration, Public Health Service, U.S. Department of Health and Human Services, December 1985).

245. Gossett, J.F., Lewis, J.M., and Barhart, F.D., *To Find A Way: The Outcome of Hospital Treatment of Disturbed Adolescents* (New York: Brunner/Mazel, 1983).

246. Gottesman, I.I., "Schizophrenia and Genetics: Where Are We? Are You Sure?" *The Nature of Schizophrenia: New Approaches to Research and Treatment*, L.C. Wynne, R.L. Cromwell, and S. Matthysse (eds.) (New York: John Wiley & Sons, 1978).

247. Gottman, J., Gonso, J., and Rasmussen, B., "Social Interaction, Social Competence and Friendship in Children," *Child Development* 46:709, 1975.

248. Gould, M.S., Wunsch-Hitzig, R., and Dohrenwend, B., "Estimating the Prevalence of Childhood Psychopathology: A Critical Review," *Journal of the American Academy of Child Psychiatry* 20:462, 1981.

249. Gray, S.W., and Klaus, R.A., "The Early Training Project: A Seventh-Year Report," *Child Development* 41:909, 1970.

250. Gray, S.W., and Wandersman, L.P., "The Methodology of Home-Based Intervention Studies: Problems and Promising Strategies," *Child Development* 51:993, 1980.

251. Graziano, A.M., and Mooney, K.C., "Family Self-Control Instruction for Children's Nighttime Fear Reduction," *Journal of Consulting and Clinical Psychology* 48:206, 1980.

252. Graziano, A.M., and Mooney, K.C., *Children and Behavior Therapy* (New York: Aldine Publishing Co., 1984).

253. Graziano, A.M., DeGiovanni, I.S., and Garcia, K.A., "Behavioral Treatment of Children's Fears: A Review," *Psychological Bulletin* 86:804, 1979.

254. Green, A.H., "Psychopathology of Abused Children," *Journal of the American Academy of Child Psychiatry* 17:92, 1978.

255. Green, A.H., "Self-Destructive Behavior in Battered Children," *American Journal of Psychiatry* 135:579, 1978.

256. Gregg, C.S., and Elmer, E., "Infant Injuries: Accident or Abuse," *Pediatrics* 44:434, 1969.

257. Grossman, H.J. (ed.), *Manual on Terminology and Classification in Mental Retardation* (Washington, DC: American Association of Mental Deficiency, 1981).

258. Group for the Advancement of Psychiatry, *Psychopathological Disorders in Childhood: Theoretical Considerations and a Proposed Classification*, Report 62 (New York: 1966).

259. Group for the Advancement of Psychiatry, *From Diagnosis to Treatment: An Approach to Treatment Planning for the Emotionally Disturbed Child*, Report 87 (New York: 1973).

260. Group for the Advancement of Psychiatry, *The Process of Child Therapy*, Report 3 (New York: Brunner/Mazel, 1982).

261. Grubb, W., *Broken Promises* (New York: Basic Books, 1982).

262. Gruenberg, E., and Huxley, J., "Mental Health Services Can Be Organized To Prevent Chronic Disability," *Community Mental Health Journal* 6:431-436, 1970.

263. Grushkin, G.M., Korsh, B.M., and Fine, R.N., "The Outlook for Adolescents With Chronic Renal Failure," *Pediatric Clinics of North America* 20:953, 1973.

264. Gualtieri, C.T., and Keppel, J.M., "Psychopharmacology in the Mentally Retarded and a Few Related Issues," *Psychopharmacology Bulletin* 21(2):304-309, 1985.

265. Guidubaldi, J., Cleminshaw, H.K., Perry, J.D., et al., "Longitudinal Effects of Divorce on Children: A Report From the NASP-KSU Nationwide Study," presented at the 92nd Annual Convention of the American Psychological Association, Toronto, Canada, August 1984.

266. Guidubaldi, J., Perry, J.D., and Clemenshaw, H.H., "The Legacy of Parental Divorce: A Na-

tionwide Study of Family Status and Selected Mediating Variables on Children's Academic and Social Competencies," *Advances in Clinical Child Psychology*, vol. 7, B.B. Lahey and A.E. Kazdin (eds.) (New York: Plenum Press, 1984).

267. Gurman, A.S., and Kniskern, D.P., "Research in Marital and Family Therapy," *Handbook of Psychotherapy and Behavior Change*, 2nd ed., S. Garfield, and A. Bergin (eds.) (New York: John Wiley & Sons, 1978).

268. Gurman, A.S., Kniskern, D.P., and Pinsof, W.M. (eds.), "Research in Marital and Family Therapy," *Handbook of Psychotherapy and Behavior Change*, 3rd ed., S. Garfield and A. Bergin (eds.) (New York: John Wiley & Sons, in press).

269. Haley, J., *Uncommon Therapy* (New York: Norton, 1973).

270. Haley, J., *Problem-Solving Therapy* (San Francisco, CA: Jossey-Bass, 1976).

271. Halmi, K.A., Falk, J.R., and Schwartz, E., "Binge-Eating and Vomiting: A Survey of a College Population," *Psychological Medicine* 11:697, 1981.

272. Hammer, M., and Kaplan, A., *The Practice of Psychotherapy With Children* (Homewood, IL: Dorsey Press, 1967).

273. Harmling, J.D., and Jones, M.B., "Birthweights of High School Dropouts," *American Journal of Orthopsychiatry* 38:63, 1968.

274. Harrison, S.I., "Individual Psychotherapy," *Comprehensive Textbook of Psychiatry, Fourth Edition*, H.I. Kaplan and B.J. Sadock (eds.) (Baltimore, MD: William & Wilkins, 1985).

275. Hartmann, D.P., Roper, B.L., and Gelfand, D.M., "An Evaluation of Alternative Modes of Child Psychotherapy," *Advances in Clinical Child Psychology*, vol. 1, B.B. Lahey and A.E. Kazdin (eds.) (New York: Plenum Press, 1977).

276. Hartstone, E., "Turnstile Children," *Corrections Today* 47:78, 1985.

277. Hartstone, E., and Cocozza, J.J., "Providing Services for the Mentally Ill, Violent Juvenile Offender," *An Anthology on Violent Juvenile Offenders*, R. Mathias, P. DeMuro, and R. Allison (eds.) (Newark, NJ: National Council on Crime and Delinquency, 1984).

277a. Harwood, H., Napolitan, D., Kristiansen, P., et al., *Economic Costs to Society of Alcohol and Drug Abuse and Mental Illness: 1980* (Research Triangle Park, NC: Research Triangle Institute, June 1984).

278. Hawton, K., and Osborn, M., "Suicide and Attempted Suicide in Children and Adolescents," *Advances in Clinical Child Psychology*, vol. 7,

B.B. Lahey and A.E. Kazdin (eds.) (New York: Plenum Press, 1984).

279. Hechtman, L., "Adolescent Outcome of Hyperactive Children Treated With Stimulants in Childhood: A Review," *Psychopharmacology Bulletin* 21(2):179, 1985.

280. Heinicke, C.M., and Strassman, L.H., "Toward More Effective Research on Child Psychotherapy," *Journal of the American Academy of Child Psychiatry* 561, 1975.

281. Heller, K., Price, R.H., and Sher, K.J., "Research and Evaluation in Primary Prevention: Issues and Guidelines," *Prevention in Mental Health: Research, Policy, and Practice*, R.H. Price, R.F. Ketterer, B.C. Bader, et al. (eds.) (Beverly Hills, CA: Sage, 1980).

282. Herrenkohl, E.C., and Herrenkohl, R.C., "A Comparison of Abused Children and Their Unabused Siblings," *Journal of the American Academy of Child Psychiatry* 18:260, 1979.

283. Herrenkohl, R.C., and Herrenkohl, E.C., "Some Antecedents and Developmental Consequences of Child Maltreatment," *New Directions for Child Development: Developmental Perspectives on Child Maltreatment*, No. 11, R. Rizley and D. Cicchetti (eds.) (San Francisco, CA: Jossey-Bass, 1981).

284. Herrenkohl, R.C., Herrenkohl, E.C., Egolf, B., et al., "The Repetition of Child Abuse: How Frequently Does It Occur?" *International Journal of Child Abuse and Neglect* 3:67, 1979.

285. Hersen, M., "The Behavioral Treatment of School Phobia," *Journal of Nervous and Mental Disease* 153:99, 1971.

286. Hersen, M., and Barlow, D.H., *Single-Case Experimental Designs: Strategies for Studying Behavioral Change* (New York: Pergamon Press, 1976).

287. Hess, R.D., "Social Class and Ethnic Influences on Socialization," *Carmichael's Manual of Child Psychology*, 3rd ed., P.H. Mussen (ed.) (New York: John Wiley & Sons, 1970).

288. Hess, R.D., and Camara, K.A., "Post-Divorce Family Relationships as Mediating Factors in the Consequences of Divorce for Children," *Journal of Social Issues* 35:79, 1979.

289. Hetherington, E.M., "Divorce: A Child's Perspective," *American Psychologist* 34:851, 1979.

290. Hetherington, E.M., and Martin, B., "Family Interaction," *Psychopathological Disorders of Childhood*, 2nd ed., H.C. Quay and J.S. Werry (eds.) (New York: John Wiley & Sons, 1979).

291. Hetherington, E.M., Cox, M., and Cox, R., "The Aftermath of Divorce," *Mother/Child, Father/*

Child Relationships, J.H. Stevens and M. Mathews (eds.) (Washington, DC: National Association for the Education of Young Children, 1978).

292. Hetherington, E.M., Cox, M., and Cox, R., "Family Interaction and the Social-Emotional and Cognitive Development of Children Following Divorce," *The Family Setting Priorities*, V. Vaughn and T. Brazelton (eds.) (New York: Science and Medicine Publishing Co., 1979).

293. Hetherington, E.M., Cox, M., and Cox, R., "Play and Social Interaction in Children Following Divorce," *Journal of Social Issues* 35:26, 1979.

294. Hetherington, E.M., Cox, M., and Cox, R., "Effects of Divorce on Parents and Children," *Nontraditional Families: Parenting and Child Development*, M.E. Lamb (ed.) (Hillsdale, NJ: Lawrence Erlbaum, 1982).

295. Higgins, J., "Effects of Child Rearing by Schizophrenic Mothers: A Followup," *Journal of Psychiatric Research* 13:1, 1976.

296. Hiscock, W.M., Chief, Child Health and Prevention Staff, Executive Office, Bureau of Program Operations, Health Care Financing Administration, U.S. Department of Health and Human Services, "FY 1985 EPSDT Program Indicators-Information," memorandum to Associate Regional Administrators, Jan. 8, 1986.

297. Hiscock, W.M., Chief, Child Health and Prevention Staff, Executive Office, Bureau of Program Operations, Health Care Financing Administration, U.S. Department of Health and Human Services, personal communication, Aug. 7, 1986.

298. Hobbs, N., *The Futures of Children: Categories, Labels, and Their Consequences* (San Francisco, CA: Jossey-Bass, 1975).

299. Hobbs, N., *Issues in the Classification of Children*, vols. 1 and 2 (San Francisco, CA: Jossey-Bass, 1975).

300. Hobbs, N., *The Troubled and Troubling Child: Re-Education in Mental Health, Education, and Human Services Programs for Children and Youth* (San Francisco, CA: Jossey-Bass, 1982).

301. Hobbs, S.A., Mogiun, L.E., Tyroler, M., et al., "Cognitive Behavior Therapy With Children: Has Clinical Utility Been Demonstrated?" *Psychological Bulletin* 87(1):147, 1980.

302. Hoffman-Plotkin, D., and Twentyman, C.T., "A Multimodal Assessment of Behavioral and Cognitive Deficits in Abused and Neglected Preschoolers," *Child Development* 55:794, 1984.

303. Horan, J.J., and Harrison, R.P., "Drug Abuse by Children and Adolescents," *Advances in Clinical Child Psychology*, vol. 4, B.B. Lahey and A.E. Kazdin (eds.) (New York: Plenum Press, 1981).

304. Horner, P., "A Continuum of Care for Juvenile Justice Clients Within a Rural Mental Health System: Program Description and Post Hoc Analysis," *Addressing the Mental Health Needs of the Juvenile Justice Population: Policies and Programs*, symposium cosponsored by the National Association of State Mental Health Program Directors and the National Institute of Mental Health, Washington, DC, Feb. 27-28, 1985.

305. Howlin, P.A., "The Effectiveness of Operant Language Training With Autistic Children," *Journal of Autism and Developmental Disorders* 11:89, 1981.

306. Huessy, H., and Cohen, A., "Hyperkinetic Behaviors and Learning Disabilities Followed Over Seven Years," *Pediatrics* 57:4, 1976.

307. Hunt, J.V., "Predicting Intellectual Disorders in Childhood for Preterm Infants With Birth Weights Below 1,501 Grams," *Preterm Birth and Psychological Development*, S.L. Friedman and M. Sigman (eds.) (New York: Academic Press, 1981).

308. Hutchinson, M.A., "Reauthorization of the Head Start Program," Testimony on Behalf of The American Psychological Association, Before the Subcommittee on Children, Family, Drugs, and Alcoholism, Senate Committee of the Labor and Human Resources, U.S. Congress, Washington, DC, Feb. 27, 1986.

309. Institute of Medicine, *Research on Mental Illness and Addictive Disorders: Progress and Prospects* (Washington, DC: National Academy Press, 1984).

310. Isaacs, M., "A Children's Mental Health Initiative: A Look at Improving the Coordination of Statewide Service Delivery Systems for Severely Emotionally Disturbed Children and Adolescents," prepared for a conference of State Mental Health Program Directors and the National Institute of Mental Health, Washington, DC, October 1983.

311. Isaacs, M.R., "A Description of 5 State Programs To Improve Service Delivery Systems for Severely Emotionally Disturbed Children and Adolescents," paper submitted to Underserved Populations Branch Office of State and Community Liaison, National Institute of Mental Health, Alcohol, Drug Abuse and Mental Health Administration, Public Health Service, U.S. Department of Health and Human Services, Rockville, MD, Aug. 30, 1983.

312. Isaacs, M.R., *A Technical Assistance Package for the Child and Adolescent Service System Pro-*

gram, vol. 1 (Rockville, MD: Office of State and Community Liaison, National Institute of Mental Health, Alcohol, Drug Abuse and Mental Health Administration, Public Health Service, U.S. Department of Health and Human Services, 1984).

313. Isaacs, Mareasa, *An Analysis of State Administrative Structures for the Provision of Coordinated Services to Children and Youth* (Bethesda, MD: Underserved Populations Branch, Office of State and Community Liaison, National Institute of Mental Health, Alcohol, Drug Abuse and Mental Health Administration, Public Health Service, U.S. Department of Health and Human Services, 1984).

314. Jagger, J., Prusoff, B.A., Cohen, D.J., et al., "The Epidemiology of Tourette's Syndrome: A Pilot Study," *Schizophrenia Bulletin* 8:267, 1982.

315. James, N.M., and Chapman, C.J., "A Genetic Study of Bipolar Affective Disorder," *British Journal of Psychiatry* 126:449, 1975.

316. Janes, C.L., Worland, J., Weeks, D.G., et al., "Interrelationships Among Possible Predictors of Schizophrenia," *Children at Risk for Schizophrenia: A Longitudinal Perspective*, N.F. Watt, E.J. Anthony, L.C. Wynne, et al. (eds.) (Cambridge, England: Cambridge University Press, 1984).

317. Jason, L.A., "A Behavioral Approach in Enhancing Disadvantaged Children's Academic Abilities," *American Journal of Community Psychology* 5:413, 1977.

318. Jason, L.A., DeAmicis, L., and Carter, B., "Preventive Intervention Programs for Disadvantaged Children," *Community Mental Health Journal* 14:272, 1978.

319. Jason, L.A., Durlak, J.A., and Holton-Walker E., "Prevention of Child Problems in the Schools," *Prevention of Problems in Childhood*, M.C. Roberts and L. Peterson (eds.) (New York: John Wiley & Sons, 1984).

320. Jencks, C.M., Smith, H., Ackland, M.B., et al., *Inequality: A Reassessment of the Effect of Family and Schooling in America* (New York: Basic Books, 1972).

321. Jessor, R., and Jessor, S.L., *Problem Behavior and Psychosocial Development; A Longitudinal Study of Youth* (New York: Academic Press, 1977).

322. Johnson, C., and Berndt, D.J. "Preliminary Investigation of Bulimia and Life Adjustment," *American Journal of Psychiatry* 140:774, 1983.

323. Johnson, M.R., "Mental Health Interventions With Medically Ill Children: A Review of the Literature," *Journal of Pediatric Psychology* 4:147, 1979.

324. Joint Commission on the Mental Health of Children, *Crisis in Child Mental Health: Challenge for the 1970's* (New York: Harper & Row, 1969).

325. Jones, C.L., Worland, J., Weeks, D.G., et al., "Interrelationships Among Possible Predictors of Schizophrenia," *Children at Risk for Schizophrenia: A Longitudinal Perspective*, N.F. Watt, E.J. Anthony, L.C. Wynne, et al. (eds.) (Cambridge, England: Cambridge University Press, 1984).

326. Kagan, S.L., Powell, D., Weiss, H.B., et al., *Family Support: The State of the Art* (New Haven, CT: Yale University Press, in press).

327. Kandel, D. (ed.), *Longitudinal Research on Drug Use: Empirical Findings and Methodological Issues* (Washington, DC: Hemisphere-Wiley, 1978).

328. Kandel, D., "Epidemiological and Psychosocial Perspectives on Adolescent Drug Use," *Journal of the American Academy of Child Psychiatry* 27:328, 1982.

329. Kanfer, F.H., Karoly, P., and Newman, A., "Reduction of Children's Fear of the Dark by Competence-Related and Situational Threat-Related Verbal Cues," *Journal of Consulting and Clinical Psychology* 43:251, 1975.

330. Kanis, J.A., Brown, P., Fitzpatrick, K., et al., "Anorexia Nervosa: A Clinical, Psychiatric, and Laboratory Study," *Quarterly Journal of Medicine* 43:321, 1974.

331. Kaplan, H.B., "Increase in Self-Rejection as an Antecedent of Deviant Responses," *Journal of Youth and Adolescence* 4(3):281, 1975.

332. Kashani, J., and Simonds, J.F., "The Incidence of Depression in Children," *American Journal of Psychiatry* 136:1203, 1979.

333. Kashani, J.H., Husain, A., Shekim, W.O., et al., "Current Perspectives on Childhood Depression: An Overview," *American Journal of Psychiatry* 138:143, 1981.

334. Katz, A.H., "Self-Help and Mutual Aid: An Emerging Social Movement?" *Annual Review of Sociology* 7:129, 1981.

335. Katzman, M.A., and Wolchik, S.A., "Bulimia and Binge Eating in College Women: A Comparison of Personality and Behavioral Characteristics," *Journal of Consulting and Clinical Psychology* 52:423, 1984.

336. Kazdin, A.E., *Treatment of Antisocial Behavior in Children and Adolescents* (Homewood, IL: Dorsey Press, 1985).

337. Kellam, S.G., Brown, C.H., and Fleming J.P., "Longitudinal Community Epidemiological Studies of Drug Use: Early Aggressiveness, Shyness, and Learning Problems," *Studying Drug Use and Abuse*, L.N. Robins (ed.) (New York: Neale Watson Academic Publications, in press).

338. Kellam, S.G., Simon, M.B., and Ensminger, M.E., Testimony in *Prevention of Drug Abuse*, Hearings Before the Select Committee on Narcotics Abuse and Control, House of Representatives, U.S. Congress (Washington, DC: U.S. Government Printing Office, April 1982).

339. Kellam, S.G., Brown, C.H., Rubin, B.R., et al., "Paths Leading to Teenage Psychiatric Symptoms and Substance Abuse: Developmental Epidemiological Studies in Woodlawn," *Childhood Psychopathology and Development*, S.B. Guze, F.J. Earls, and J.E. Barrett (eds.) (New York: Raven Press, 1983).

340. Kendall, P.C., "Cognitive-Behavioral Interventions With Children," *Advances in Clinical Child Psychology*, vol. 4, B.B. Lahey and A.E. Kazdin (eds.) (New York: Plenum Press, 1981).

341. Kendall, P.C., and Braswell, L., *Cognitive-Behavioral Therapy for Impulsive Children* (New York: Guilford Press, 1985).

342. Kendall, P.C., and Zupan, B.A., "Individual Versus Group Application of Cognitive Behavioral Strategies for Developing Self-Control in Children," *Behavior Therapy* 12:344, 1981.

343. Kennedy, W.A., "School Phobia: Rapid Treatment of Fifty Cases," *Journal of Abnormal Psychology* 70:285, 1965.

344. Kent, J.T., "A Followup Study of Abused Children," *Journal of Pediatric Psychology* 1:25, 1976.

345. Khantzian, E.J., "An Ego/Self Theory of Substance Dependence: A Contemporary Psychoanalytic Perspective," *Theories in Drug Abuse*, NIDA Research Monograph 30, No. ADM 80-967, D.J. Lettieri, D. Sayers, and H.W. Pearson (eds.) (Rockville, MD: National Institute on Drug Abuse, Alcohol, Drug Abuse, and Mental Health Administration, Public Health Service, U.S. Department of Health and Human Services, 1980).

346. Kiesler, C.A., "Public and Professional Myths About Mental Hospitalization: An Empirical Reassessment of Policy-Related Beliefs," *American Psychologist* 37:12, 1982.

347. Kifer, R.E., Lewis, M.A., Green, D.R., et al., "Training Predelinquent Youths and Their Parents To Negotiate Conflict Situations," *Journal of Applied Behavior Analysis* 7:357, 1974.

348. Kinard, E.M., "Emotional Development in Physically Abused Children," *American Journal of Orthopsychiatry* 50:686, 1980.

349. Kinard, E.M., and Klerman, L.V., "Teenage Parenting and Child Abuse: Are They Related?" *American Journal of Orthopsychiatry* 50(3):481, 1980.

350. Kinney, J.M., Madsen, B., Fleming, T., et al., "Homebuilders: Keeping Families Together," *Journal of Consulting and Clinical Psychology* 45(4):667, 1977.

351. Kirkland, K.D., and Thelen, M.H., "Uses of Modeling in Child Treatment," *Advances in Clinical Child Psychology*, vol. 1, B.B. Lahey and A.E. Kazdin (eds.) (New York: Plenum Press, 1977).

352. Kirschner Associates, *A National Survey of the Impacts of Head Start Centers on Community Institutions*, ED 045195 (Albuquerque, NM: 1970).

353. Klein, J.I., "The Least Restrictive Alternative: More About Less," *Psychiatry 1982: American Psychiatric Association Annual Review*, L. Grinsporn (ed.) (Washington, DC: American Psychiatric Press, 1982).

354. Klein, L., "Early Teenage Pregnancy, Contraception and Repeat Pregnancy," *American Journal of the Diseases of Children* 122:15, 1971.

355. Klein, M., and Stern, L., "Low Birth Weight and the Battered Child Syndrome," *American Journal of the Diseases of Children* 122:15, 1971.

356. Klein, N.C., Alexander, J.F., and Parsons, B.V., "Impact of Family Systems Intervention on Recidivism and Sibling Delinquency: A Model of Primary Prevention and Program Evaluation," *Journal of Consulting and Clinical Psychology* 45:469, 1977.

357. Klerman, G.L., "Age and Clinical Depression: Today's Youth in the 21st Century," *Journal of Gerontology* 31(3):318, 1976.

358. Knitzer, J., *Unclaimed Children* (Washington, DC: Children's Defense Fund, 1982).

359. Knitzer, J., "Developing Systems of Care for Disturbed Children: The Role of Advocacy," unpublished paper, Institute for Child and Youth Policy Studies, Rochester, NY, 1984.

360. Kohn, M.L., *Class and Conformity: A Study in Values* (Homewood, IL: Dorsey Press, 1969).

361. Kohut, H., *The Restoration of the Self* (New York: International Universities Press, 1977).

362. Kolvin, I., Garside, R.F., Nicol, A.R., et al., *Help Starts Here: The Maladjusted Child in the Ordinary School* (London, England: Tavistock Publications, 1981).

363. Koocher, G., and Broskowski, A., "Issues in the Evaluation of Mental Health Services for Children," *Professional Psychology* 8:583, 1977.

364. Koocher, G.P., and O'Malley, J.E., *The Damocles Syndrome* (New York: McGraw Hill, 1981).

365. Koocher G.P., and Pedulla, B.M., "Current Practices in Child Psychotherapy," *Professional Psychology* 8:275, 1977.

366. Koski, M.A., and Ingram, E.M., "Child Abuse and Neglect: Effects on Bayley Scale Scores," *Journal of Abnormal Child Psychology* 5:79, 1977.

367. Kovacs, M., and Beck, A.T., "Maladaptive Cognitive Structures in Depression," *American Journal of Psychiatry* 135:525, 1978.

368. Kresler, C.A., "Public and Professional Myths About Mental Hospitalization: An Empirical Reassessment of Policy-Related Beliefs," *American Psychologist* 37:1325, 1982.

369. Krug, R.S., "Substance Abuse," *Handbook of Clinical Child Psychology*, C.E. Walker and M.C. Roberts (eds.) (New York: John Wiley & Sons, 1983).

370. Kurdek, L.A., "An Integrative Perspective on Children's Divorce Adjustment," *American Psychologist* 36:855, 1981.

371. Kuyler, P., Rosenthal, L., Igel, G., et al., "Psychopathology Among Children of Manic Depressive Patients," *Biological Psychiatry* 15:589, 1980.

372. Lacayo, N., Sherwood, G., and Morris, J., "Daily Activities of School Psychologists: A National Survey," *Psychology in the Schools* 18:184, 1981.

373. Landis, J.T., "Experiences of 500 Children With Adult Sexual Deviation," *Psychiatric Quarterly Supplement* 30:91, 1956.

374. Lang, A., "State Laws Mandating Private Health Insurance Benefits for Mental Health, Alcoholism, and Drug Abuse," *State Health Reports*, No. 20, January 1986.

375. Langsley, D.G., and Kaplan, D.M., *Treatment of Families in Crisis* (New York: Grune & Stratton, 1968).

376. Laurenitis, L.R., "Psychotherapy and Social Skills Training for the Learning Disabled," presented at the 92nd Annual Convention of the American Psychological Association, Toronto, Ontario, August 1984.

377. Lauer, B., Broeck, E., and Grossman, M., "Battered Child Syndrome: Review of 130 Patients With Controls," *Pediatrics* 54:67, 1974.

378. Lazar, I., and Darlington, R., "Lasting Effects of Early Education: A Report From the Consortium for Longitudinal Studies," *Monographs of the Society for Research in Child Development*, Serial No. 195, 47:2 (Chicago, IL: University of Chicago Press for the Society for Research in Child Development, 1982).

379. Leckman, J.F., Detlor, J., and Cohen, D.J., "Gilles de la Tourette Syndrome: Emerging Areas of Clinical Research," *Childhood Psychopathology and Development*, S.B. Guze, F.J. Earls, and J.E. Barrett (eds.) (New York: Raven Press, 1983).

380. Lee, E.E., "Alcohol Education and the Elementary School Teacher," *The Journal of School Health* 46:271, 1976.

381. Leon, C.M.D., McKnew, D.H., Zahn-Waxler, et al., "A Developmental View of Affective Disturbances in the Children of Affectively Ill Parents," *American Journal of Psychology* 141(2):219, 1984.

382. Levitt, E.E., "The Results of Psychotherapy With Children: An Evaluation," *Journal of Consulting Psychology* 21(3):189, 1957.

383. Levitt, E.E., "Psychotherapy With Children: A Further Evaluation," *Behavioral Research and Therapy* 1:45, 1963.

384. Lewis, D.O., Lewis, M., Unger, L., et al., "Conduct Disorder and Its Synonyms: Diagnosis of Dubious Validity and Usefulness," *American Journal of Psychiatry* 141:514, 1984.

385. Lewis, M., Feiring, C., McGuffog, G., et al., "Predicting Psychopathology in Six-Year-Olds From Early Social Relations," *Child Development* 55:123, 1984.

386. Lewis, M., Lewis, D.O., Shanok, S.S., et al., "The Undoing of Residential Treatment," *Journal of Child Psychiatry* 19:168, 1980.

387. Light, R.J., and Pillemer, D.B., *Summing Up: The Science of Reviewing Research* (Cambridge, MA: Harvard University Press, 1984).

388. Lindemann, E., "Symptomatology and Management of Acute Grief," *American Journal of Psychiatry* 101:141, 1944.

389. Links, P.S., "Community Survey of the Prevalence of Childhood Psychiatric Disorders: A Review," *Child Development* 54:531, 1983.

390. Lipman, R.S., DiMascio, A., Reatig, N., et al., "Psychotropic Drugs and Mentally Retarded Children," *Psychopharmacology: A Generation of Progress*, M.A. Lipton, A. DiMascio, and K. Killam (eds.) (New York: Raven Press, 1978).

391. Lipsett, L.P., "Perinatal Risks, Neonatal Deficits, and Developmental Crisis," *Preterm Birth and Psychological Development*, S.L. Friedman and M. Sigman (eds.) (New York: Academic Press, 1981).

392. Loehlin, J.C., Lindzey, G., and Spuhler, J.N., *Race Differences in Intelligence* (San Francisco, CA: Freeman, 1975).

393. Lorenzi, M.E., Klerman, L.V., and Jekel, J.F., "School-Age Parents: How Permanent a Relationship?" *Adolescence* 45:13, 1977.

394. Lorion, R.P., Caldwell, R.A., and Cowen, E.L.,

"Effects of a School Mental Health Project: A One-Year Follow-Up," *Journal of School Psychology* 14:56, 1976.

395. Loughran, E.J., "The Juvenile Justice System and Mental Health: A Juvenile Justice Perspective," *Addressing the Mental Health Needs of the Juvenile Justice Population: Policies and Programs*, symposium cosponsored by the National Association of State Mental Health Program Directors and the National Institute of Mental Health, Washington, DC, Feb. 27-28, 1985.

396. Lourie, I., and Katz-Leavy, J., "Severely Emotionally Disturbed Children," presented at the National Conference on Chronic Patients II, Kansas City, KS, August 1984.

397. Lourie, I., Fishman, M., Hersh, S., et al., *Chronically Mentally Ill Children and Adolescents: A Special Report for the National Plan for the Chronically Mentally Ill* (Rockville, MD: National Institute of Mental Health, Alcohol, Drug Abuse, and Mental Health Administration, Public Health Service, U.S. Department of Health and Human Services, 1980).

398. Lovaas, O.I., "Parents as Therapists," *Autism: A Reappraisal of Concepts and Treatment*, M. Rutter and E. Schopler (eds.) (New York: Plenum Press, 1978).

399. Luria, A.R., *The Role of Speech in the Regulation of Normal and Abnormal Behavior* (New York: Liveright, 1961).

400. Lutzker, J.R., "Deviant Family Systems," *Advances in Clinical Child Psychology*, vol. 3, B.B. Lahey and A.E. Kazdin (eds.) (New York: Plenum Press, 1980).

401. Lynch, M., and Roberts, J., "Predicting Child Abuse: Signs of Bonding Failure in the Maternity Hospital," *British Medical Journal* 1(6061): 624, 1977.

402. Madanes, C., "Protection, Paradox, and Pretending," *Family Process* 19:73, 1980.

403. Magrab, P.R., Sostek, A.M., and Powell, B.A., "Prevention in the Prenatal Period," *Prevention of Problems in Childhood*, M.C. Roberts and L. Peterson (eds.) (New York: John Wiley & Sons, 1984).

404. Mahler, M.S., and Furer, M., "Child Psychosis: A Theoretical Statement and Its Implications," *Journal of Autism and Childhood Schizophrenia* 2(3):213, 1972.

405. Manderscheid, R.W. and Witkin, M.J., "The Specialty Mental Health Services Delivery System-United States," Alcohol, Drug Abuse, and Mental Health Administration, Public Health Service, U.S. Department of Health and Human Services, *Mental Health, United States 1983*,

C.A. Taube and S.A. Barrett (eds.), DHHS Pub. No. (ADM)83-1275 (Washington, DC: U.S. Government Printing Office, 1983).

406. Manderscheid, R., Witkin, M., Rosenstein, M., et al., "Specialty Mental Health Services: System and Patient Characteristics-United States," Alcohol, Drug Abuse, and Mental Health Administration, Public Health Service, U.S. Department of Health and Human Services, *Mental Health, United States, 1985*, G.A. Taube and S.A. Barrett (eds.) (Washington, DC: U.S. Government Printing Office, 1985).

407. Mannarino, A.P., and Durlak, J.A., "Implementation and Evaluation of Services Programs in Community Settings," *Professional Psychology* 11:220, 1980.

408. Mannino, F.V., and Shore, M.F., "The Effects of Consultation: A Review of Empirical Studies," *American Journal of Community Psychology* 3(1):1, 1975.

409. Marecek, J., *Economic, Social and Psychological Consequences of Adolescent Childbearing: An Analysis of Data From the Philadelphia Collaborative Perinatal Project*, final report to National Institute of Child Health and Human Development, National Institutes of Health, Public Health Service, U.S. Department of Health and Human Services, Washington, DC, September 1979.

410. Margolies, P.J., "Behavioral Approaches to the Treatment of Early Infantile Autism: A Review," *Psychological Bulletin* 84:249, 1977.

411. Marsden, G., McDermott, J.F., and Miner, D., "Residential Treatment of Children: A Survey of Institutional Characteristics," *Journal of the American Academy of Child Psychiatry* 9:332, 1970.

412. Marsden, G., McDermott, J.F., and Miner, D., "Selection of Children for Residential Treatment," *Journal of the American Academy of Child Psychiatry* 16:423, 1977.

413. Martin, H.P., "The Child and His Development," *Helping the Battered Child and His Family*, C.H. Kenpe and R.E. Helfer (eds.) (Philadelphia, PA: Lippincott, 1972).

414. Martin, H.P., and Beezley, P., "Personality of Abused Children," *The Abused Child*, H.P. Martin (ed.) (Cambridge, MA: Ballinger, 1976).

415. Martin, H.P., and Beezeley, P., "Behavioral Observations of Abused Children," *Developmental Medicine and Child Neurology* 19:373, 1977.

416. Martin, H.P., Beezley, P., Conway, E., et al., "The Development of Abused Children," *Advances in Pediatrics* 21:25, 1974.

417. Marton, P., Minde, K., and Oglivie, J., "Mother-

Infant Interactions in the Premature Nursery," *Preterm Birth and Psychological Development*, S.L. Friedman and M. Sigman (eds.) (New York: Academic Press, 1981).

418. Mash, E.J., and Terdal, L.G. (eds.), *Behavioral Assessment of Childhood Disorders* (New York: Guilford Press, 1981).

419. Massimo, J.L., and Shore, M.F., "The Effectiveness of a Comprehensive, Vocationally Oriented Psychotherapeutic Program for Adolescent Delinquent Boys," *American Journal of Orthopsychiatry* 33:634, 1963.

420. Masterpasqua, F., and Swift, M., "Prevention of Problems in Childhood on a Community-Wide Basis," *Prevention of Problems in Childhood*, M.C. Roberts and L. Peterson (eds.) (New York: John Wiley & Sons, 1984).

421. Matas, L., Arend, R., and Sroufe, L.A., "Continuity in Adaptation in the Second Year," *Child Development* 49:547, 1978.

422. Matson, J.L., "Emotional Problems in the Mentally Retarded: The Need for Assessment and Treatment," *Psychopharmacology Bulletin* 21(2): 258, 1985.

423. Mattson, A., "Long-Term Physical Illness in Childhood: A Challenge to Psychosocial Adaptation," *Pediatrics* 50:801, 1972.

424. McAdoo, W.G., and DeMyer, M.K., "Personality Characteristics of Parents," *Autism: A Reappraisal of Concepts and Treatment,* M. Rutter and E. Schopler (eds.) (New York: Plenum Press, 1978).

425. McAnarney, E.R., Pless, I.B., Satterwhite, B., et al., "Psychological Problems of Children With Chronic Juvenile Arthritis," *Pediatrics* 53:523, 1974.

426. McIsaac, B.C., "Integration of Cognitive and Affective Intervention," paper presented at the annual convention of the American Psychological Association, Toronto, Ontario, 1984.

427. McKenry, P.C., Walters, L.H., and Johnson, C., "Adolescent Pregnancy: A Review of the Literature," *The Family Coordinator* 28:17, 1979.

428. McKnew, D., Cytryn, L., Efron, A., et al., "Offspring of Patients With Affective Disorders," *British Journal of Psychiatry* 134:148, 1979.

429. McMahon, R.J., and Forehand, R., "Self-Help Behavior Therapies in Parent Training," *Advances in Clinical Child Psychology*, vol. 3, B.B. Lahey and A.E. Kazdin (eds.) (New York: Plenum Press, 1980).

430. McNeil, T.F., and Kaij, L., "Offspring of Women With Nonorganic Psychoses," *Children at Risk for Schizophrenia: A Longitudinal Perspective*, N.F. Watt, E.J. Anthony, L.C. Wynne, et al. (eds.) (Cambridge, England: Cambridge University Press, 1984).

431. Mednick, S.A., Cudek, R., Griffith, J.J., et al., "The Danish High-Risk Project: Recent Methods and Findings," *Children at Risk for Schizophrenia: A Longitudinal Perspective*, N.F. Watt, E.J. Anthony, L.C. Wynne, et al. (eds.) (Cambridge, England: Cambridge University Press, 1984).

432. Meeks, J.E., "Conduct Disorders," *Comprehensive Textbook of Psychiatry*, H.I. Kaplan and B.J. Saddock (eds.) (Baltimore, MD: William & Wilkins, 1980).

433. Meichenbaum, D., and Goodman, J., "Training Impulsive Children to Talk to Themselves: A Means of Developing Self-Control," *Journal of Abnormal Psychology* 77:115, 1971.

434. Meisels, S., "Prediction, Prevention, and Developmental Screening in the EPSDT Program," *Child Development Research and Social Policy*, H.W. Stevenson and A.E. Siegel (eds.) (Chicago, IL: University of Chicago Press, 1984).

435. Mendelson, W., Johnson, N., and Stewart, M.A., "Hyperactive Children as Teenagers: A Followup Study," *Journal of Nervous Mental Disorders* 153:273, 1971.

436. Messer, S.B., "Reflection-Impulsivity: A Review," *Psychological Bulletin* 83:1026, 1976.

437. Meyers, J., Parson R.D., and Martin, R., *Mental Health Consultation in the School* (San Francisco, CA: Jossey-Bass, 1979).

438. Meyers, J.C., "Federal Efforts To Improve Mental Health Services for Children: Breaking a Cycle of Failure," unpublished paper, University of Michigan, Ann Arbor, MI, 1985.

439. Milich, R., and Loney, J., "The Role of Hyperactive and Aggressive Symptomatology in Predicting Adolescent Outcome Among Hyperactive Children," *Journal of Pediatric Psychology* 4:93, 1979.

440. Miller, F.J.W., Court, S.D.M., Walton, W.S., et al., *Growing Up in Newcastle-Upon-Tyne* (London, England: Oxford University Press, 1960).

441. Minde, K., Weiss, G., and Mendelson, B., "A Five-Year Followup Study of 91 Hyperactive School Children," *Journal of the American Academy of Child Psychiatry* 11:595, 1972.

442. Minuchin, S., *Families and Family Therapy* (Cambridge, MA: Harvard University Press, 1974).

443. Minuchin, S., Rosman, B., and Baker, L., *Psychosomatic Families* (Cambridge, MA: Harvard University Press, 1978).

444. Minuchin, S., Barker, L., Rosman, B., et al., "A Conceptual Model of Psychosomatic Illness in

Children," *Archives of General Psychiatry* 32:1031, 1975.

445. Minuchin, S., Montalvo, B., Gverney, B., et al., *Families of the Slums* (New York: Basic Books, 1967).

446. Monkus, E., and Bancalari, E., "Neonatal Outcome," *Teenage Parents and Their Offspring*, K.G. Scott, T. Field, and E.G. Robertson (eds.) (New York: Grune & Stratton, 1981).

447. Morgan, S.R., "Psychoeducational Profile of Emotionally Disturbed Abused Children," *Journal of Clinical Psychology* 8:3, 1979.

448. Morse, C.W., Sahler, O.J., and Friedman, S.B., "A Three-Year Followup Study of Abused and Neglected Children," *American Journal of Diseases in Children* 120:439, 1970.

449. Moscowitz, I.S., "The Effectiveness of Day Hospital Treatment; A Review," *Journal of Community Psychology* 8:155, 1980.

450. Mowrer, O.H., "Apparatus for the Study and Treatment of Enuresis," *American Journal of Psychology* 51:163, 1938.

451. Mrazek, P.B., "Sexual Abuse of Children," *Advances in Clinical Child Psychology*, vol. 6, B.B. Lahey and A.E. Kazdin (eds.) (New York: Plenum Press, 1983).

452. Mrazek, P.B., and Mrazek, D.A., "The Effects of Child Sexual Abuse: Methodological Considerations," *Sexually Abused Children and Their Families*, P.B. Mrazek and C.H. Kempe (eds.) (Oxford, England: Pergamon Press, 1981).

453. Mrazek, P.B., Lynch, M., and Bentovim, A., "Recognition of Child Sexual Abuse in the United Kingdom," *Sexually Abused Children and Their Families*, P.B. Mrazek and C.H. Kempe (eds.) (Oxford, England: Pergamon Press, 1981).

454. Mumford, E., Schlesinger, H.J., Glass, G.V., et al., "A New Look at Evidence About Reduced Costs of Medical Utilization Following Mental Health Treatment," *American Journal of Psychiatry* 141(10):1145, 1984.

455. Namir, S., and Weinstein, R.S., "Children: Facilitating New Directions," *Reaching the Underserved: Mental Health Needs of Neglected Populations: Sage Annual Reviews of Community Mental Health*, vol. 3, L.R. Snowden (ed.) (Beverly Hills, CA: Sage, 1982).

456. National Academy of Sciences, *Making Policies for Children* (Washington, DC: National Academy Press, 1982).

457. National Association of Private Psychiatric Hospitals, *The Annual Survey 1984 Results* (Washington, DC: 1984).

458. National Association of Private Psychiatric Hospitals, *The Annual Survey 1985 Results* (Washington, DC: 1985).

459. National Association of State Mental Health Program Directors, *Funding Sources and Expenditures for State Mental Health Agencies: Fiscal Year 1983* (Washington, DC: 1985).

460. Neale, J.M., Winters, K.C., and Weintraut, S., "Information Processing Deficits in Children at High Risk for Schizophrenia," *Children at Risk for Schizophrenia: A Longitudinal Perspective*, N.F. Watt, E.J. Anthony, L.C. Wynne, et al. (eds.) (Cambridge, England: Cambridge University Press, 1984).

461. Needleman, H.L., and Bellinger, D., "The Developmental Consequences of Childhood Exposure to Lead," *Advances in Clinical Child Psychology*, vol. 7, B.B. Lahey and A. Kazdin (eds.) (New York: Plenum Press, 1984).

462. Neeper, R., and Lahey B.B., "Learning Disabilities of Children," *Handbook of Clinical Child Psychology*, C.E. Walker and M.E. Roberts (eds.) (New York: John Wiley & Sons, 1983).

463. Newlund, S., "Appeals Court Medicaid Ruling Could Aid Mental Patient Funding," *Detroit Free Press*, Sept. 30, 1983, p. R-11.

464. Nurnberger, J.I., and Gershon, E.S., "Genetics," *Handbook of Affected Disorders*, E.S. Paykel (ed.) (New York: Guilford Press, 1982).

465. O'Connell, M., and Moore, M., "The Legitimacy Status of First Births to U.S. Women Aged 15-24, 1939-1978," *Family Planning Perspectives* 12(1):16, 1980.

466. O'Connell, M., and Rogers, C.C., "Out-of-Wedlock Births, Premarital Pregnancies and Their Effect in Family Formation and Dissolution," *Family Planning Perspectives* 16(4), 1984.

467. O'Connell, R.A., Mayo, J.A., O'Brien, J.D., et al., "Children of Bipolar Manic-Depressives," *The Genetics of Affective Disorder*, J. Mendlewicz and B. Shopsin (eds.) (New York: Spectrum Publications, 1979).

468. O'Dell, S., "Training Parents in Behavior Modification: A Review," *Psychological Bulletin* 81(7): 418, 1974.

469. O'Keefe, A., *What Head Start Means to Families*, Administration for Children, Youth, and Families, Office of Human Development Services, U.S. Department of Health, Education, and Welfare, DHEW Pub. No. (OHDS) 79-31129 (Washington, DC: U.S. Government Printing Office, 1979).

470. O'Leary, K.D., "Etiology of Hyperactivity: A

Social Learning Analysis," presented at the Convention of the American Psychological Association in Toronto, Canada, Aug. 24, 1984.

471. O'Leary, K.D., and Johnson, S.B., "Psychological Assessment," *Psychopathological Disorders of Childhood,* 2nd ed., H.C. Quay and J.S. Werry (eds.) (New York: John Wiley & Sons, 1979).

472. O'Leary, K.D., and Turkewitz, N., "Methodological Errors in Marital and Child Treatment Research," *Journal of Consulting and Clinical Psychiatry* 46:797, 1978.

473. O'Leary, K.D., Pelham, W.E., Rosenbaum, A., et al., "Behavioral Treatment of Hyperkinetic Children," *Clinical Pediatrics* 15:510, 1976.

474. O'Malley, T.E., Koocher, G., Foster, D., et al., "Psychiatric Sequelae of Surviving Childhood Cancer," *American Journal of Orthopsychiatry* 49:608, 1979.

475. Orbach, S., "Visibility/Invisibility: Social Considerations in Anorexia Nervosa—A Feminist Perspective," *Theory and Treatment of Anorexia and Bulimia: Biomedical, Sociocultural, and Psychological Perspectives,* S.W. Emmett (ed.) (New York: Brunner/Mazel, 1985).

476. Orvaschel, H., "Parental Depression and Child Psychopathology," *Childhood Psychopathology and Development,* S.B. Guze, F.J. Earls, and J.E. Barrett (eds.) (New York: Raven Press, 1983).

477. Orvaschel, H., Weissman, M.M., Padian, N., et al., "Assessing Psychopathology in Children of Psychiatrically Disturbed Parents," *Journal of the American Academy of Child Psychiatry* 20:112, 1981.

478. Osofsky, H., "Poverty, Pregnancy Outcome, and Child Development," *Birth Defects* 10:37, 1974.

479. Ounstead, C., Oppenheimer, R., and Lindsay, J., "Aspects of Bonding Failure: The Psychopathology and Psychotherapeutic Treatment of Families of Battered Children," *Developmental Medicine and Child Neurology* 16:447, 1974.

480. Owens, A., "Why Pyschiatrists' Earnings Aren't Keeping Up," *Medical Economics,* April 1986, pp. 174-179.

481. Palmer, J., *The Psychological Assessment of Children* (New York: John Wiley & Sons, 1970).

482. Palmer, T., "The Youth Authority's Community Treatment Project," *Federal Probation* 38:3, 1974.

483. Pandina, R.J., and Schuele, J.A., "Psychosocial Correlates of Alcohol and Drug Use of Adolescent Students and Adolescents in Treatment," *Journal of Studies on Alcohol* 44(6):950, 1983.

484. Parloff, M., "Can Psychotherapy Research Guide the Policy Makers: A Little Knowledge May Be a Dangerous Thing," *American Psychologist* 34:296, 1979.

485. Parsons, B.V., and Alexander, J.F., "Short-Term Family Intervention: A Therapy Outcome Study," *Journal of Consulting and Clinical Psychology* 41:195, 1973.

486. Paton, S., Kessler, R., and Kandel, D., "Depressive Mood and Adolescent Illicit Drug Use: A Longitudinal Analysis," *Journal of Genetic Psychology* 131:267, 1977.

487. Patterson, G.R., "Interventions for Boys With Conduct Problems: Multiple Settings, Treatment and Criteria," *Journal of Consulting and Clinical Psychology* 42(4):471, 1974.

488. Patterson, G.R., "Retraining of Aggressive Boys by Their Parents: Review of Recent Literature and Followup Evaluations," *Canadian Psychiatric Association Journal* 19:142, 1974.

489. Patterson, G.R., *Living With Children* (Champaign, IL: Research Press, 1976).

490. Patterson, G.R., "Parents and Teachers as Change Agents: Social Rearing Approach System," *Treating Relationships,* D.M.L. Olson (ed.) (Lake Mills, IA: Graphic Publishing, 1976).

491. Patterson, G.R., "The Aggressive Child: Victim and Architect of a Coercive System," *Behavior Modification and Families,* L.A. Hamerlynck, E.J. Mash, and L.C. Handy (eds.) (New York: Brunner/Mazel, 1976).

492. Patterson, G.R., and Cobb, J.A., "A Dyadic Analysis of 'Aggressive' Behaviors," *Minnesota Symposia on Child Psychology,* vol. 5., J.P. Hill (ed.) (Minneapolis, MN: University of Minnesota Press, 1971).

493. Patterson, G.R., and Fleischmann, M.J., "Maintenance of Treatment Effects: Some Considerations Concerning Family Systems and Followup Data," *Behavior Therapy* 10:168, 1979.

494. Patterson, G.R., and Reid, J.B., "Intervention for Families of Aggressive Boys: A Replication Study," *Behavior Research and Therapy* 11:383, 1973.

495. Patterson, G.R., Chamberlain, P., and Reid, J.B., "A Comparative Evaluation of a Parent-Training Program," *Behavior Therapy* 13:638, 1982.

496. Patterson, G.R., Cobb, J.A., and Ray, R.S., "A Social Engineering Approach for Retraining Families of Aggressive Boys," *Issues and Trends in Behavior Therapy,* H. Adams and I. Unikel (eds.) (Springfield, IL: Charles C. Thomas, 1973).

497. Patterson, G.R., Reid, J.B., Jones, R.R., et al.,

A Social Learning Approach to Family Intervention, vol. 1 (Eugene, OR: Castalia Press, 1975).

498. Paulson, G., Rizvi, A., and Crane, G., "Tardive Dyskinesia as a Possible Sequel of Long-Term Therapy With Phenothiazines," *Clinical Pediatrics* 14:953, 1975.

499. Pelton, L.H., "Child Abuse and Neglect: The Myth of Classlessness," *American Journal of Orthopsychiatry* 48:608, 1978.

500. Pelton, L.H., *The Social Context of Child Abuse and Neglect* (New York: Human Sciences Press, 1981).

501. Perris, C., "A Study of Bipolar and Unipolar Recurrent Depressive Psychoses," *Acta Psychiatrica Scandinavica* 42:68, 1966.

502. Perry, M.A., Doran, L., and Wells, E.A., "Developmental and Behavioral Characteristics of the Abused Child," *Journal of Clinical Child Psychology* 12:320, 1983.

503. Persons, R.W., "Relationship Between Psychotherapy With Institutionalized Boys and Subsequent Community Adjustment," *Journal of Consulting Psychology* 31:137, 1967.

504. Peterson, L., and Ridley-Johnson, R., "Prevention of Disorders in Children," *Handbook of Clinical Child Psychology*, C.E. Walker and M.C. Roberts (eds.) (New York: John Wiley & Sons, 1983).

505. Petti, T.A., "Depression in Hospitalized Child Psychiatry Patients: Approaches to Measuring Depression," *Journal of the American Academy of Child Psychiatry* 17:49, 1978.

506. Pfeffer, C.R., "Suicidal Behavior of Children: A Review With Implications for Research and Practice," *American Journal of Psychiatry* 138:154, 1981.

507. Pfeifer, G.D., and Weinstick-Savoy, D., "Peer Culture and the Organization of Self and Object Representations in Children's Psychotherapy Groups," *Social Work With Groups* 7(4):39, 1984.

508. Philips, I., "Childhood Depression: Interpersonal Interactions and Depression Phenomenon," *American Journal of Psychiatry* 136:511, 1979.

509. Philips, I., and Williams, N., "Psychopathology and Mental Retardation: A Study of One Hundred Mentally Retarded Children: I Psychopathology," *American Journal of Psychiatry* 132:1265, 1975.

510. Piaget, J., *The Language and Thought of the Child* (New York: Harcourt Brace, 1926).

511. Pless, I.B., and Roghmann, K.J., "Chronic Illness and Its Consequences: Observations Based on Three Epidemiologic Surveys," *Journal of Pediatrics* 79:351, 1971.

512. Polivy, J., and Herman, P.C., "Dieting and Binging: A Causal Analysis," *American Psychologist* 40(2):193, 1985.

513. Pops, M., and Schwabe, A.D., "Hypercarotenemia in Anorexia Nervosa," *Journal of the American Medical Association* 205:533, 1968.

514. President's Commission on Mental Health, *Report to the President From the President's Commission on Mental Health*, vol. 1 (Commission Report) and vol. 3 (Task Panel Reports) (Washington, DC: U.S. Government Printing Office, 1978).

515. Prior, M., "Developing Concepts of Childhood Autism: The Influence of Experimental Cognitive Research," *Journal of Consulting and Clinical Psychology* 52:4, 1984.

516. Provence, S., Naylor, A., and Patterson, J., *The Challenge of Daycare* (New Haven, CT: Yale University Press, 1977).

517. Puig-Antich, J., "Major Depression and Conduct Disorder in Prepuberty," *Journal of the American Academy of Child Psychiatry* 21(2):118, 1982.

518. Puig-Antich, J., Ryan, N., and Rabinovich, H., "Affective Disorders in Childhood and Adolescence," *Diagnosis and Psychopharmacology of Childhood and Adolescent Disorders*, J.M. Wiener (ed.) (New York: John Wiley & Sons, 1985).

519. Puig-Antich, J., Novacenko, H., Davies, M., et al., "Growth Hormone Secretion in Prepubertal Children With Major Depression," *Archives of General Psychiatry* 45:455, 1984.

520. Quay, H.C., "Classification," *Psychopathological Disorders of Childhood*, H.C. Quay and J.S. Werry (eds.) (New York: John Wiley & Sons, 1979).

521. Quay, H.C., "Residential Treatment," *Psychopathological Disorders of Childhood*, H.C. Quay and J.S. Werry (eds.) (New York: John Wiley & Sons, 1979).

522. Quint, J.C., and Riccio, J.A., *The Challenge of Serving Pregnant and Parenting Teens: Lessons From Project Redirection* (New York: Manpower Demonstration Research Corp., April 1985).

523. Quinton, D., and Rutter, M., "Early Hospital Admissions and Later Disturbances of Behavior: An Attempted Replication of Douglas' Findings," *Developmental Medicine and Childhood Neurology* 18:447, 1976.

524. Ramey, C.T., commentary in I. Lazar and R. Darlington, "Lasting Effects of Early Education: A Report From the Consortium for Longitudinal Studies," *Monographs of the Society for Research in Child Development*, vol. 47, Nos. 2-3, 1982.

525. Ramey, C.T., MacPhee, D., and Yeates, K.O., "Preventing Developmental Retardation: A General Systems Model," *Facilitating Infant and Early Childhood Development*, L.A. Bond and J.M. Jaffe (eds.) (Hanover, NH: University Press of New England, 1982).

526. Rapoport, J.L., "Stimulant Drug Treatment of Hyperactivity: An Update," *Childhood Psychopathology and Development*, S.B. Guze, F.J. Earls, and J.E. Barnett (eds.) (New York: Raven Press, 1983).

527. Rapoport, J.L., and Mikkelsen, E.J., "Antidepressants," *Pediatric Psychopharmacology: The Use of Behavior Modifying Drugs in Children*, J.S. Werry (ed.) (New York: Brunner/Mazel, 1978).

528. Rapoport, J.L., Quinn, P., Bradbard, G., et al., "Imipramine and Methylphenidate Treatments of Hyperactive Boys," *Archives of General Psychiatry* 30:789, 1974.

529. Redfering, D.L., "Group Counseling With Institutionalized Delinquent Females," *American Corrective Therapy Journal* 26:160, 1972.

530. Redfering, D.L., "Durability of Effects of Group Counseling With Institutionalized Delinquent Females," *Journal of Abnormal Psychology* 82:85, 1973.

531. Redick, R.W., and Witkin, M.J., "Residential Treatment Centers for Emotionally Disturbed Children, United States, 1977-78 and 1979-80," *Mental Health Statistical Note No. 162*, DHHS Pub. No. (ADM) 83-158 (Rockville, MD: National Institute of Mental Health, Alcohol, Drug Abuse, and Mental Health Administration, Public Health Service, U.S. Department of Health and Human Services, 1983).

532. Regier, D.A., Goldberg, I.D., and Taube, C.A., "The De Facto U.S. Mental Health Services System," *Archives of General Psychiatry* 35:685, 1978.

533. Regier, D.A., Myers, J.K., Kramer, M., et al., "The NIMH Epidemiologic Catchment Area Program: Historical Context, Major Objectives, and Study Population Characteristics," *Archives of General Psychiatry* 41:934, 1984.

534. Reidy, T.J., "The Aggressive Characteristics of Abused and Neglected Children," *Journal of Clinical Psychology* 33:1140, 1977.

535. Reidy, T.J., Anderegg, T.R., Tracy, R.J., et al., "Abused and Neglected Children: The Cognitive, Social and Behavioral Correlates," *Traumatic Abuse and Neglect of Children at Home*, G.J. Williams and J. Meney (eds.) (Baltimore, MD: Johns Hopkins Press, 1980).

536. Reisinger, J.J., and Lavigne, J.V., "An Early Intervention Model for Pediatric Settings," *Professional Psychology* 11:582, 1980.

537. Reisman, J., *Principles of Psychotherapy With Children* (New York: John Wiley & Sons, 1973).

538. Reiss, S., Levitan, G.W., and McNally, R.J., "Emotionally Disturbed Mentally Retarded People: An Underserved Population," *American Psychologist* 37(4):361, 1982.

539. Rescola, L.A., Provence, S., and Naylor, A., "The Yale Child Welfare Research Program: Description and Results," *Day Care: Scientific and Social Policy Issues*, E.F. Zigler and E.W. Gordon (eds.) (Boston, MA: Auburn, 1982).

540. Richard, H.C., Elkins, P.D., "Behavior Therapy With Children," *Handbook of Clinical Child Psychology*, C.E. Walker and M.C. Roberts (eds.) (New York: John Wiley & Sons, 1983).

541. Rider, R.V., Taback, M., and Knobloch, H., "Associations Between Premature Births and Socioeconomic Status," *American Journal of Public Health* 45:1022, 1955.

542. Robbins, D.R., and Alessi, N.E., "Depressive Symptoms and Suicidal Behavior in Adolescents," *American Journal of Psychiatry* 142:588, 1985.

543. Roberts, M.C., and Wright, L., "The Role of the Pediatric Psychologist as Consultant to Pediatricians," *Handbook for the Practice of Pediatric Psychology*, J. Tuma (ed.) (New York: Wiley-Interscience, 1982).

544. Robins, L.N., *Deviant Children Grown Up* (Baltimore, MD: Williams & Wilkins, 1966).

545. Robins, L.N., "Sturdy Childhood Predictors of Adult Antisocial Behavior: Replications From Longitudinal Studies," *Psychological Medicine* 8:611, 1978.

546. Robins, L.N., "Follow-up Studies of Behavior Disorders in Children," *Psychopathological Disorders in Childhood*, 2nd ed., H.C. Quay and J.S. Werry (eds.) (New York: John Wiley & Sons, 1979).

547. Robins, L.N., Davis, D.H., and Wish, E., "Detecting Predictors of Rare Events: Demographic, Family, and Personal Deviance as Predictors of Stages in the Progression Toward Narcotic Addiction," *The Origins and Course of Psychopathology: Methods of Longitudinal Research*, J.S. Strauss, H. Babigian, and M. Roff (eds.) (New York: Plenum Press, 1977).

548. Rodriguez, A.R., "Psychological and Psychiatric Peer Review at CHAMPUS," *American Psychologist* 38(8):941, 1983.

549. Rodriguez, A.R., "Peer Review Program Sets Trends in Claims Processing," *Business and Health* 21, 1984.

550. Rolf, J.E., "The Social and Academic Competence of Children Vulnerable to Schizophrenia and Other Behavior Pathologies," *Journal of Abnormal Psychology* 80:225, 1972.

551. Rolf, J.E., and Garmezy, N., "The School Performance of Children Vulnerable to Behavior Pathology," *Life History Research in Psychopathology*, vol. 3, M. Roff (ed.) (Minneapolis, MN: University of Minnesota Press, 1974).

552. Rosenthal, R., *Meta-Analytic Procedures for Social Research*, Applied Social Research Methods Series, vol. 6 (Beverly Hills, CA: Sage, 1984).

553. Ross, A.O., *Psychological Disorders of Children: A Behavioral Approach to Theory, Research and Therapy* (New York: McGraw-Hill, 1980).

554. Ross, A.O., and Nelson, R.O., "Behavior Therapy," *Psychopathological Disorders of Childhood*, 2nd ed., H.C. Quay and J.S. Werry (eds.) (New York: John Wiley & Sons, 1979).

555. Ross, A.O., and Pelham, W.E., "Child Psychopathology," *Annual Review of Psychology* 32: 243, 1981.

556. Ross, D., and Ross, S., *Hyperactivity: Research, Theory and Action* (New York: McGraw-Hill, 1976).

557. Ruby, G., "New Health Professionals in Child and Maternal Health," *Better Health for Our Children: A National Strategy*, vol. 4, background papers (Washington, DC: U.S. Department of Health and Human Services, 1981).

558. Rudd, L., "Pregnancies and Abortions," *Self-Destructive Behavior in Children and Adolescents*, C.F. Wells and I.R. Stuart (eds.) (New York: Van Nostrand Reinhold Co., 1981).

559. Russell, M., Henderson, C., and Blume, S.B., *Children of Alcoholics: A Review of the Literature* (New York: Children of Alcoholics Foundation, 1984).

560. Rutter, M., *Children of Sick Parents: An Environmental and Psychiatric Study* (London, England: Oxford University Press, 1966).

561. Rutter, M., "Psychological Therapies: Issues and Prospects," *Childhood Psychopathology and Development*, S.B. Guze, F.J. Earls, and J.E. Barrett (eds.) (New York: Raven Press, 1983).

562. Rutter, M., and Graham, P., "Psychiatric Disorder in 10- and 11-Year-Old Children," *Proceedings of the Royal Society of Medicine* 59: 382, 1966.

563. Rutter, M., and Shaffer, D., "DSM-III: A Step Forward or Back in Terms of the Classification of Child Psychiatric Disorders?" *Journal of the American Academy of Child Psychiatry* 19:371-394, 1980.

564. Rutter, M., Tizard, J., and Whitmore, K., *Education, Health and Behavior* (London, England: Longman Group, Ltd., 1970).

565. Rutter, M., Yule, W., and Graham, P., "Enuresis and Behavioral Deviance: Some Epidemiological Considerations," *Bladder Control and Enuresis*, I. Kolvin, R. MacKeith, and S.R. Meadow (eds.) (London, England: SIMP Heinemann, 1973).

566. Rutter, M., Cox, A., Tupling, C., et al., "Attainment and Adjustment in Two Geographical Areas. I. Prevalence of Psychiatric Disorder," *British Journal of Psychiatry* 126:493, 1975.

567. Safer, D.J., and Krager, J.M., "Prevalence of Medication Treatment for Hyperactive Adolescents," *Psychopharmacology Bulletin* 21(2):212, 1985.

568. Safer, R., and Allen, D., *Hyperactive Children: Diagnosis and Management* (Baltimore, MD: University Park Press, 1976).

569. Sameroff, A.J., "Longitudinal Studies of Preterm Infants," *Preterm Births and Psychological Development*, S.L. Friedman and M. Sigman (eds.) (New York: Academic Press, 1981).

570. Sameroff, A.J., and Chandler, M.J., "Reproductive Risk and the Continuum of Caretaking Casualty," *Review of Child Development Research*, vol. 4, F.D. Horowitz (ed.) (Chicago, IL: University of Chicago Press, 1975).

571. Sameroff, A.J., Barocas, R., and Seifer, R., "The Early Development of Children Born to Mentally Ill Women," *Children at Risk for Schizophrenia: A Longitudinal Perspective*, N.F. Watt, E.J. Anthony, L.C. Wynne, et al. (eds.) (Cambridge, England: Cambridge University Press, 1984).

572. Sameroff, A.J., Seifer, R., and Zax, M., "Early Development of Children at Risk for Emotional Disorders," *Monographs of the Society for Research in Child Development* 47:7 (Chicago, IL: University of Chicago Press for the Society for Research in Child Development, 1982).

573. Sandler, H.M., *Effects of Adolescent Pregnancy on Mother-Infant Relationships: A Transactional Model*, progress reports to National Institute of Child Health and Human Development, Washington, DC, June 1977, January 1978, May 1978, and June 1979.

574. Sarason, I.G., and Ganzer, V.J., "Modeling and Group Discussion in the Rehabilitation of Juvenile Delinquents," *Journal of Counseling Psychology* 20:442, 1973.

575. Sarason, S.B., "Community Psychology and Public Policy: Missed Opportunity," *American Journal of Community Psychology* 12:199, 1984.

576. Sattler, J.M., *Assessment of Children's Intelli-*

gence and Special Abilities, 2nd ed. (Boston, MA: Allyn & Bacon, 1982).

577. Satterfield, J., Satterfield, B., and Cantwell, D., "Three Year Multimodality Treatment Study of 100 Hyperactive Boys," Journal of Pediatrics 98:650, 1981.

578. Sauber, M., "Life Situations of Mothers Where First Child Was Born Out of Wedlock," Illegitimacy: Changing Services for Changing Lives (New York: National Council on Illegitimacy, 1970).

579. Saxe, L., and Dougherty, D., "Technology Assessment and Congressional Use of Social Psychology: Making Complexity Useful," Applied Social Psychology Annual, vol. 4, S. Oskamp (ed.) (Beverly Hills, CA: Sage, in press).

580. Saxe, L., and Fine, M., Social Experiments (Beverly Hills, CA: Sage, 1981).

581. Saxe, L., Dougherty, D., and Esty, K., "The Effectiveness and Cost of Alcoholism Treatment: A Public Policy Perspective," The Diagnosis and Treatment of Alcoholism, J.H. Mendelson, and N.K. Mello (eds.) (New York: McGraw-Hill, 1985).

582. Schamess, G., "Group Treatment Modalities for Latency-Age Children," International Journal of Group Psychotherapy 26:455, 1976.

583. Schmitt, B., and Kempe, H., "Neglect and Abuse of Children," Nelson Textbook of Pediatrics, V. Vaughan and R. McKay (eds.) (Philadelphia, PA: Saunders, 1975).

584. Schneider-Rosen, K., and Cicchetti, D., "The Relationship Between Affect and Cognition in Maltreated Infants: Quality of Attachment and the Development of Self-Recognition," Child Development 55:648, 1984.

585. Schopler, E., and Reichler, R.J., "Parents as Cotherapists in the Treatment of Psychotic Children," Journal of Autism and Childhood Schizophrenia 1:87, 1971.

586. Schroeder, S.R., and Gualtieri, C.T., "Behavioral Interactions Induced by Chronic Neuroleptic Therapy in Persons With Mental Retardation," Psychopharmacology Bulletin 21(2):310, 1985.

587. Schulman, J.L., and Irwin, M., Psychiatric Hospitalization of Children (Springfield, IL: Charles C. Thomas, 1982).

588. Schurman, R.A., Kramer, P.D., and Mitchell, J.B., "The Hidden Mental Health Network: Treatment of Mental Illness by Nonpsychiatrist Physicians," Archives of General Psychiatry 42(1):89-94, 1985.

589. Schwartz, I.M., "The Youth Element in Health Care-Costs," Minnesota Journal 1(2):1, 1983.

590. Schwartz, I.M., testimony of Ira M. Schwartz on behalf of the Hubert H. Humphrey Institute of Public Affairs, University of Minnesota, before the U.S. House of Representatives Select Committee on Children, Youth and Families, Washington, DC, June 6, 1985.

591. Schwitzgebel, R.L., "Preliminary Socialization for Psychotherapy of Behavior Disordered Adolescents," Journal of Consulting and Clinical Psychology 33:71, 1969.

592. Scott, K.G., Field, T., Robertson, E.G., et al. (eds.), Teenage Parents and Their Offspring (New York: Grune & Stratton, 1981).

593. Seidel, U.P., Chadwick, O.F.D., and Rutter, M., "Psychological Disorders in Crippled Children: A Comparative Study of Children With and Without Brain Damage," Developmental Medicine and Child Neurology 17:563, 1975.

594. Seitz, V., Rosenbaum L.K., and Apfel, N.H., "Effects of Family Support Intervention: A Ten-Year Follow-Up," Child Development 56:376, 1985.

595. Select Panel for the Promotion of Child Health, Better Health for Our Children: A National Strategy, presented to the U.S. Congress and the Secretary of Health and Human Services, Washington, DC, 1981.

596. Shaffer, D., Gardner, A., and Hedge, B., "A Critical Examination of Classification Systems of Nocturnal Enuresis," Childhood Psychopathology and Development, S.B. Guze, F.J. Earls, and J.E. Barrett (eds.) (New York: Raven Press, 1983).

597. Shafii, M., McCue, A., Ice, J.F., et al., "The Development of an Acute Short-Term Inpatient Child Psychiatric Setting: A Pediatric-Psychiatric Model," American Journal of Psychiatry 136:(4a), 1979.

598. Shapiro, A.K., Shapiro, E., Brunn, R.D., et al., Gilles de la Tourette Syndrome (New York: Raven Press, 1978).

599. Shapiro, S., Skinner, E.A., Kessler, L.G., et al., "Utilization of Health and Mental Health Services," Archives of General Psychiatry 41:971-978, October 1984.

600. Sharfstein, S.S., Muszynski, S., and Myers, E., Health Insurance and Psychiatric Care: Update and Appraisal (Washington, DC: American Psychiatric Press, Inc., 1984).

601. Shore, M.F., "The Mental Health System and Juvenile Justice: A Mental Health Perspective," Addressing the Mental Health Needs of the Juvenile Justice Population: Policies and Programs, symposium cosponsored by the National Association of State Mental Health Program Direc-

tors and the National Institute of Mental Health, Washington, DC, Feb. 27-28, 1985.

602. Shore, M.F., and Mannino, F.V., "Mental Health Services for Children and Youth," *Journal of the Clinical Child Psychology* 5(3):21, 1976.

603. Shore, M.F., and Massimo, J., "Comprehensive Vocationally Oriented Psychotherapy for Adolescent Boys: A Followup Study," *American Journal of Orthopsychiatry* 36:609, 1966.

604. Shore, M.F., and Massimo, J.L., "Five Years Later: A Followup Study of Comprehensive Vocationally Oriented Psychotherapy," *American Journal of Orthopsychiatry* 39(5):769, 1969.

605. Shore, M.F., and Massimo, J.L., "After Ten Years: A Followup Study of Comprehensive Vocationally Oriented Psychotherapy," *American Journal of Orthopsychiatry* 43(1):128, 1973.

606. Short, M.J., Kirby, T., and Wilson, C.T., "A Followup Study of Disturbed Children Treated in a Re-ED Program," *Hospital and Community Psychiatry* 28(9):694, 1977.

607. Siegal, L.S., "The Prediction of Possible Learning Disabilities in Preterm and Full-Term Children," *Infants Born at Risk*, T. Field and A. Sostek (eds.) (New York: Grune & Stratton, 1983).

608. Sills, J., Thomas, L., and Rosenbloom, L., "Non-Accidental Injury: A Two-Year Study in Central Liverpool," *Developmental Medicine and Child Neurology* 19:26, 1977.

609. Silver, L.B., "Chronic Mental Illness in Children and Adolescents: Scope of the Problem," paper for the National Conference on Chronic Mental Illness in Children and Adolescents, sponsored by the American Psychiatric Association, Dallas, TX, March 1985.

610. Simons, B., Downs, E.F., Hurster, M.M., et al., "Child Abuse: Epidemiologic Study of Medically Reported Cases," *New York State Journal of Medicine* 66:2783, 1966.

611. Skinner, B.F., *Behavior of Organisms: An Experimental Analysis* (New York: Appleton-Century-Crofts, 1938).

612. Skynner, A.C.R., "An Open-Systems, Group Analytic Approach to Family Therapy," *Handbook of Family Therapy*, A.S. Gurman and D.P. Kniskern (eds.) (New York: Brunner/Mazel, 1981).

613. Smeraldi, E., Negri, F., and Melicaam, A., "A Genetic Study of Affective Disorder," *Acta Psychiatrica Scandinavica* 56:382, 1977.

614. Smetana, J.G., Kelly, M., and Twentyman, C.T., "Abused, Neglected, and Non-Maltreated Children's Conceptions of Moral and Social-Conventional Transgressions," *Child Development* 55:277, 1984.

615. Smith, G.M., and Fogg, C.P., "Psychological Predictors of Early Use, Late Use, and Nonuse of Marijuana Among Teenage Students," *Longitudinal Research on Drug Use: Empirical Findings and Methodological Issues*, D.B. Kandel (ed.) (Washington, DC: Hemisphere-Wiley, 1978).

616. Smith, G.M., Glass, G.V., and Miller, T.J., *The Benefits of Psychotherapy* (Baltimore, MD: Johns Hopkins University Press, 1980).

617. Smith, S., Hanson, R., and Noble, S., "Social Aspects of the Battered Baby Syndrome," *British Journal of Psychiatry* 125:568, 1974.

618. Solnit, A.J., Cohen, D., Anders, T., et al., "Childhood Disorders," unpublished background paper for Institute of Medicine, National Academy of Sciences, *Research on Mental Illness and Addictive Disorders: Progress and Prospects* (Washington, DC: National Academy Press, 1984).

619. Sowder, B.J. (ed.), "Community Mental Health Services for Children: Recent Experiences and Future Planning," summary of *The Proceedings of a Workshop on Community Mental Health Services for Children*, prepared under Order No. PLD-06951-77RC, final report, Sept. 22, 1977.

620. Spack, N.P., "Medical Complications of Anorexia Nervosa and Bulimia," *Theory and Treatment of Anorexia and Bulimia; Biomedical, Sociocultural, and Psychological Perspectives*, S.W. Emmett (ed.) (New York: Brunner/Mazel, 1985).

621. Spivack, C., Platt, J.J., and Shure, M.B., *The Problem Solving Approach to Adjustment* (San Francisco, CA: Jossey-Bass, 1976).

622. Sprague, R.L., "Principles of Clinical Trials and Social, Ethical and Legal Issues of Drug Use in Children," *Pediatric Psychopharmacology: The Use of Behavior Modifying Drugs in Children*, J.S. Werry (ed.) (New York: Brunner/Mazel, 1978).

623. Sroufe, L.A., "Infant-Caregiver Attachment and Patterns of Adaptation in Preschool: The Roots of Maladaptation and Competence," *Minnesota Symposium in Child Psychology*, vol. 16, M. Perlmutter (ed.) (Minneapolis, MN: University of Minnesota Press, 1983).

624. Stewart, M.A., Cummings, C., Singer, S., et al., "The Overlap Between Hyperactive and Unsocialized Aggressive Children," *Journal of Child Psychology and Psychiatry* 22:35, 1981.

625. Stone, L.A., "Residential Treatment," *Basic Handbook of Child Psychiatry*, vol. 3, J.D. Noshpitz (ed.) (New York: Basic Books, 1979).

626. Strangler, R.S., and Printz, A.M., "DSM-III: Psychiatric Diagnosis in a University Popula-

tion," *American Journal of Psychiatry* 137:937, 1980.

627. Sugar, M., "Infants of Adolescent Mothers: Research Perspectives," *Adolescent Parenthood*, M. Sugar (ed.) (New York: Spectrum Publications, 1984).

628. Swanson, J.M., and Kinsbourne, M., "Stimulant-Related State-Dependent Learning in Hyperactive Children," *Science* 192:1354, 1976.

629. Swift, C.R., and Seidman, F.L., "Adjustment Problems of Juvenile Diabetes," *Journal of the American Academy of Child Psychiatry* 3:500, 1964.

630. Tanguary, P.E., "Toward a New Classification of Serious Psychopathology in Children," *Journal of the American Academy of Child Psychiatry* 23(4):373, 1984.

631. Task Force on the Commitment of Minors, "Guidelines for the Psychiatric Hospitalization of Minors," *American Journal of Psychiatry* 139(7): 971, 1982.

632. Taube, C., Lee, E.S., and Forthofer, R.N., "Diagnosis-Related Groups for Mental Disorders, Alcoholism and Drug Abuse: Evaluation and Alternatives," *Hospital and Community Psychiatry* 35(5):452, 1984.

632a. Taube, C. and Rupp, A., "The Effect of Medicaid on Access to Ambulatory Mental Health Care for the Poor and Near-Poor Under 65," *Medical Care* 24(8):677, August 1986.

633. Tavormina, J.B., Kastner, L.S., Slater, P.M., et al., "Chronically Ill Children—A Psychologically and Emotionally Deviant Population," *Journal of Abnormal Child Psychology* 4:99, 1976.

634. Terr, L.C., "A Family Study of Child Abuse," *American Journal of Psychiatry* 127:125, 1970.

635. Thompson, T., and Reynolds, J., "The Results of Intensive Care Therapy for Neonates: I. Overall Neonatal Mortality Rates, II. Neonatal Mortality Rates and Long-Term Prognosis for Low Birth Weight Neonates," *Journal of Perinatal Medicine* 5:59, 1977.

636. Toff, Gail E., *Mental Health Benefits Under Medicaid: A Survey of the States* (Washington, DC: Intergovernmental Health Policy Project, George Washington University, 1984).

637. Tramontana, M.G., "Critical Review of Research in Psychotherapeutic Outcomes With Adolescents, 1967-1973," *Psychological Bulletin* 88:429, 1980.

638. Trickett, D.K., Apfel, N.H., Rosenbaum L.K., et al., "A Five-Year Followup of Participants in the Yale Child Welfare Research Program," *Day Care: Scientific and Social Policy Issues*, E.F. Zigler and E.W. Cordon (eds.) (Boston, MA: Auburn, 1982).

639. Trieschman, A.E., Whittaker, J.U., and Brendtro, C.K., *The Other Twenty-Three Hours* (Chicago, IL: Aldine, 1969).

640. Tulkin, S.R., and Kagan, J., "Mother-Child Interaction in the First Year of Life," *Child Development* 43:31, 1972.

641. Turkington, C., "Aversive Therapy: Report Faulting Institute Refuels Debate on Its Use," *APA Monitor* 17(6):24, June 1896.

642. Ungerer, J.A., and Sigman, M., "Developmental Lags in Preterm Infants From One to Three Years of Age," *Child Development* 54:1217, 1983.

643. Urbain, E.S., and Kendall, P.C., "Review of Social Cognitive Problem Solving Interventions With Children," *Psychological Bulletin* 88(1): 109, 1980.

643a. U.S. Congress, General Accounting Office "Defense Health Programs: Changes in Administration of Mental Health Benefits," fact sheet for the Honorable Daniel K. Inouye, United States Senate (Gaithersburg, MD: U.S. General Accounting Office, June 1986).

643b. U.S. Congress, General Accounting Office, *States Have Made Few Changes In Implementing The Alcohol, Drug Abuse, And Mental Health Services*, HRD-8452 (Washington, DC: U.S. Government Printing Office, June 6, 1984).

644. U.S. Congress, House of Representatives, Committee on Ways and Means, *Children in Poverty* (Washington, DC: U.S. Government Printing Office, 1985).

645. U.S. Congress, House of Representatives, Select Committee on Children, Youth, and Families, "Opportunities for Success: Cost-Effective Programs for Children," staff report (Washington, DC: U.S. Government Printing Office, August 1985).

646. U.S. Congress, Library of Congress, Congressional Research Service, "Summary of Poor Children: A Study of Trends and Policy, 1968-1984," presented to the Subcommittee on Public Assistance and Unemployment Compensation, Committeee on Ways and Means, House of Representatives, U.S. Congress, Washington, DC, May 22, 1985.

647. U.S. Congress, Office of Technology Assessment, *The Efficacy and Cost-Effectiveness of Psychotherapy*, OTA-HCS-18 (Washington, DC: U.S. Government Printing Office, 1980).

648. U.S. Congress, Office of Technology Assessment, *The Effectiveness and Costs of Alcoholism Treatment*, OTA-HCS-22 (Washington, DC: U.S. Government Printing Office, March 1983).

649. U.S. Congress, Office of Technology Assessment, *Medicare's Prospective Payment Plan: Strategies for Evaluating Cost, Quality, and*

Medical Technology, OTA-H-262 (Washington, DC: U.S. Government Printing Office, October 1985).

650. U.S. Congress, Senate Committee on the Judiciary, Subcommittee on Juvenile Justice, *A Hearing on Teenage Suicide*, hearing Oct. 3, 1984 (Washington, DC: U.S. Government Printing Office, 1984).

651. U.S. Department of Commerce, Bureau of the Census, Washington, DC, unpublished data for 1969, 1975, 1980.

652. U.S. Department of Commerce, Bureau of the Census, *Marital Status and Living Arrangements, March 1981 (Current Population Reports)* (Washington, DC: U.S. Government Printing Office, 1982).

653. U.S. Department of Defense, *Psychiatric Care: Cost and Utilization Under Civilian Health and Medical Program of the Uniformed Services (CHAMPUS)* (Washington, DC: U.S. Government Printing Office, 1983).

654. U.S. Department of Defense, "Civilian Health and Medical Program of the Uniformed Services (CHAMPUS): Treatment of Mental Disorders," *Federal Register* 49(180):36087, 1984.

655. U.S. Department of Defense, Office of Civilian Health and Medical Program of the Uniformed Services, Statistics Branch, "Estimated Cost-Savings Resulting From the 60-Day Limitation on Inpatient Psychiatric Care in CY 1983," CHAMPUS Management Information Report, OMIR 85-01 (Aurora, CO: April 1985).

656. U.S. Department of Education, Office of Special Education and Rehabilitative Services, Division of Educational Services, Special Education Programs, "Abstract: Survey of Expenditures for Special Education and Related Services," Washington, DC, no date.

657. U.S. Department of Education, Office of Special Education and Rehabilitative Services, Division of Educational Services, Special Education Programs, *To Assure the Free Appropriate Public Education of All Handicapped Children*, Seventh Annual Report to Congress on the Implementation of the Education of the Handicapped Act, Washington, DC, 1985.

658. U.S. Department of Health, Education, and Welfare, Project on the Classification of Exceptional Children, *Report of the Conference on the Use of Stimulant Drugs in the Treatment of Behaviorally Disturbed Young School Children* (Washington, DC: Development, 1971).

659. U.S. Department of Health, Education, and Welfare, Office of Human Development Services, National Center on Child Abuse and Neglect, *Child Sexual Abuse: Incest, Assault and Sexual Exploitation*, DHEW Pub. No. 79-30166 (Washington, DC: 1978).

660. U.S. Department of Health and Human Services, Health Care Financing Administration, *Medicare and Medicaid Data Book* (Washington, DC: June 1986).

661. U.S. Department of Health and Human Services, Health Care Financing Administration, Bureau of Program Operations, Grants Branch, Division of State Agency Financial Management, unpublished data pertaining to fiscal year 1985 Medicaid program expenditure information, BPO-F31, Baltimore, MD, September 1986.

661a. U.S. Department of Health and Human Services, National Center for Health Services Research and Health Care Technology Assessment, *Private Health Insurance in the United States,* National Health Care Expenditures Study Data Preview 23, DHHS Pub. No. (PHS)86-3406 (Rockville, MD: September 1986).

662. U.S. Department of Health and Human Services, Office of Human Development Services, Administration for Children, Youth and Families, Children's Bureau, National Center on Child Abuse and Neglect, *Study Findings: National Study of Incidence and Severity of Child Abuse and Neglect*, DHHS Pub. No. 81-03025 (OHDS) (Washington, DC: September 1981).

663. U.S. Department of Health and Human Services, Public Health Service, Alcohol, Drug Abuse, and Mental Health Administration, National Institute of Mental Health, *Mental Health, United States, 1983*, C.A. Taube and S.A. Barrett (eds.), DHHS Pub. No. (ADM) 83-1275 (Rockville, MD: 1983).

664. U.S. Department of Health and Human Services, Public Health Service, Alcohol, Drug Abuse, and Mental Health Administration, National Institute of Mental Health, *Eleventh Annual Report on the Child and Youth Activities* (Rockville, MD: 1984).

665. U.S. Department of Health and Human Services, Public Health Service, Alcohol, Drug Abuse, and Mental Health Administration, National Institute of Mental Health, *Mental Health, United States, 1985*, C.A. Taube and S.A. Barrett (eds.), DHHS Pub. No. (ADM) 85-1378 (Rockville, MD: 1985).

666. U.S. Department of Health and Human Services, Public Health Service, Alcohol, Drug Abuse, and Mental Health Administration, National Institute of Mental Health, *Network Analysis Methods for Mental Health Service System Research: A Comparison of Two Community Support Systems*, Mental Health Service System Reports, Series BN No. 6, J.P. Morrissey, et al. (eds.),

DHHS Pub. No. (ADM) 85-1383 (Rockville, MD: 1985).

667. U.S. Department of Health and Human Services, Public Health Service, Alcohol, Drug Abuse, and Mental Health Administration, National Institute of Mental Health, "Responses to 1983 Inventory of Mental Health Organizations," unpublished, Rockville, MD, February 1986.

668. U.S. Department of Health and Human Services, Public Health Service, Alcohol, Drug Abuse, and Mental Health Administration, National Institute of Mental Health, *Twelfth Annual Report on the Child and Youth Activities of the National Institute of Mental Health, Federal Fiscal Year 1985*, report to the National Advisory Mental Health Council by M.E. Fishman, Mar. 10, 1986 (Rockville, MD: 1986).

668a. U.S. Department of Health and Human Services, Public Health Service, Alcohol, Drug Abuse, and Mental Health Administration, National Institute of Mental Health and U.S. Department of Justice, Office of Juvenile Justice and Deliquency Prevention, *Juvenile Offenders With Serious Drug, Alcohol, and Mental Health Problems, Executive Summary* (Rockville, MD: ADAMHA, 1986).

669. U.S. Department of Health and Human Services, Public Health Service, National Center for Health Statistics, "Advance Report of Final Natality Statistics, 1981," *Monthly Vital Statistics Report* 32(9):supp., 1983.

670. U.S. Department of Health and Human Services, Public Health Service, National Center for Health Statistics, "Utilization and Expenditures for Ambulatory Mental Health Care During 1980," *National Medical Care Utilization and Expenditure Survey, Data Report No. 5*, DHHS Pub. No. (PHS) 84-20000 (Washington, DC: U.S. Government Printing Office, June 1984).

671. Valentine, J., and Stark, E., "The Social Context of Parent Involvement in Head Start," *Project Head Start: A Legacy of the War on Poverty*, E. Zigler and J. Valentine (eds.) (New York: Free Press, 1979).

672. Varley, C.K., "A Review of Studies of Drug Treatment Efficacy With Attention Deficit Disorder With Hyperactivity in Adolescents," *Behavioral Pediatrics* 98(4):650, 1981.

673. Varley, C.K., "A Review of Studies of Drug Treatment Efficacy for Attention Deficit Disorder With Hyperactivity in Adolescents," *Psychopharmacology Bulletin* 21(2):216, 1985.

674. Vygotsky, L.S., *Thought and Language* (New York: John Wiley & Sons, 1962).

675. Waldron, S., "The Significance of Childhood Neurosis for Adult Mental Health," *American Journal of Psychiatry* 133:532, 1976.

676. Wallerstein, J.S., and Kelly, J.B., "The Effects of Parental Divorce: The Adolescent Experience," *The Child and His Family*, vol. 3, E. Anthony and C. Koupernik (ed.) (New York: John Wiley & Sons, 1974).

677. Wallerstein, J.S., and Kelly, J.B., "The Effects of Parental Divorce: Experiences of the Preschool Child," *Journal of the American Academy of Child Psychiatry* 19:600, 1975.

678. Wallerstein, J.S., and Kelly, J.B., "The Effects of Parental Divorce: Experiences of the Child in Later Latency," *American Journal of Orthopsychiatry* 46:256, 1976.

679. Wallerstein, J.S., and Kelly, J.B., "California's Children of Divorce," *Psychology Today* 13(8):66, 1980.

680. Wallerstein, J.S., and Kelly, J.B., *Surviving the Breakup: How Children and Parents Cope With Divorce* (New York: Basic Books, 1980).

681. Walter, H.I., and Gilmore, S.K., "Placebo Versus Social Learning Effects in Parent Training Procedures Designed To Alter the Behavior of Aggressive Boys," *Behavior Therapy* 4:361, 1973.

682. Watt, N.F., "In a Nutshell: The First Two Decades of High-Risk Research in Schizophrenia," *Children at Risk for Schizophrenia: A Longitudinal Perspective*, N.F. Watt, E.J. Anthony, L.C. Wynne, et al. (eds.) (Cambridge, England: Cambridge University Press, 1984).

683. Watt, N.F., Grobb, T.W., and Erlenmeyer-Kimling, L., "Social, Emotional, and Intellectual Behavior at School Among Children at High Risk for Schizophrenia," *Children at Risk for Schizophrenia: A Longitudinal Perspective*, N.F. Watt, E.J. Anthony, L.C. Wynne, et al. (eds.) (Cambridge, England: Cambridge University Press, 1984).

684. Watzlawick, P., Weakland, J., and Fish, R., *Change: Principles of Problem Formation and Problem Resolution* (New York: Norton, 1979).

685. Wegscheider, D., and Wegscheider, S., *Family Illness: Chemical Dependency* (Crystal, MN: Nurturing Works, 1978).

686. Weinstein, L., *Evaluation of a Program for Re-Education Disturbed Children: A Followup Comparison With Untreated Children* (Washington, DC: U.S. Department of Health, Education, and Welfare, 1974).

687. Weintraub, S., and Neale, J.M., "Social Behavior of Children at Risk for Schizophrenia," *Children*

at Risk for Schizophrenia: A Longitudinal Perspective, N.F. Watt, E.J. Anthony, L.C. Wynne, et al. (eds.) (Cambridge, England: Cambridge University Press, 1984).

688. Weintraub, S., Neale, J.M., and Liebert, D.E., "Teacher Ratings of Children Vulnerable to Psychopathology," *American Journal of Orthopsychiatry* 5:839, 1975.

689. Weintraub, S., Prinz, R.J., and Neale, J.M., "Peer Evaluations of the Competence of Children Vulnerable to Psychopathology," *Journal of Abnormal Child Psychology* 4:461, 1978.

690. Weintrob, A., "Long-Term Treatment of the Severely Disturbed Adolescent: Residential Treatment Versus Hospitalization," *Journal of the American Academy of Child Psychiatry* 14:436, 1975.

691. Weiss, B., "Food Additive Safety Evaluation: The Link to Behavioral Disorders in Children," *Advances in Clinical Child Psychology*, vol. 7, B.B. Lahey and A.E. Kazdin (eds.) (New York: Plenum Press, 1984).

692. Weiss, G., Minde, K., Werry, J.S., et al., "Studies on the Hyperactive Child. VIII. Five Year Followup," *Archives of General Psychiatry* 24:409, 1971.

693. Weiss, H.B., "Introduction in Family Support Project and Family Resource Coalition," *Programs To Strengthen Families: A Resource Guide* (New Haven, CT: Yale University Press, 1983).

694. Weissberg, R.P., Cowen, E.L., Lotyezewski, B.S., et al., "The Primary Mental Health Project (PMHP): Seven Consecutive Years of Program Outcome Research," *Journal of Consulting and Clinical Psychology* 51:100, 1983.

695. Weissman, M.M., and Klerman, G.L., "Sex Differences in the Epidemiology of Depression," *Archives of General Psychiatry* 35:1304, 1977.

696. Weissman, M.M., Paykel, E.S., and Klerman, G.L., "The Depressed Woman as a Mother," *Social Psychiatry* 7:98, 1972.

697. Weissman, M.M. Prusoff, B.A., Gammon, G.D., et al., "Psychopathology in the Children of Depressed and Normal Parents," *Journal of the American Academy of Child Psychiatry* 23:78, 1984.

698. Wender, P.H., Wood, D.R., and Reimherr, F.W., "Pharmacological Treatment of Attention Deficit Disorder, Residual Type (ADD,RT 'Minimal Brain Dysfunction,' 'Hyperactivity' in Adults)," *Psychopharmacological Bulletin* 21(2):222, 1985.

699. Werner, E., and Smith, R.S., *Kauai's Children Come of Age* (Honolulu, HI: University of Hawaii Press, 1977).

700. Werry, J.S., "The Childhood Psychoses," *Psy-*

chopathological Disorders of Childhood, H.C. Quay and J.S. Werry (eds.) (New York: John Wiley & Sons, 1979).

701. Werry, J.S., "Psychosomatic Disorders, Psychogenic Symptoms and Hospitalization," *Psychopathological Disorders of Childhood*, H.C. Quay and J.S. Werry (eds.) (New York: John Wiley & Sons, 1979).

702. Werry, J.S., and Quay, H.C., "The Prevalence of Behavior Symptoms in Younger Elementary School Children," *American Journal of Orthopsychiatry* 41:136, 1971.

703. West, D.J., and Farrington, D.P., *Who Becomes Delinquent?* (London, England: Heinemann Educational, 1973).

704. Whitaker, C.A., and Keith, D.V., "Symbolic-Experimental Family Therapy," *Handbook of Family Therapy*, A.S. Gurman and D.P. Kniskern (eds.) (New York: Brunner/Mazel, 1981).

705. Whitt, J.K., "Children's Adaptation to Chronic Illness and Handicapping Conditions," *Chronic Illness and Disability Through the Life Span: Effects on Self and Family*, M.G. Eisenberg, L.C. Sutkin, and M.A. Jansen (eds.) (New York: Springer, 1984).

706. Whittaker, J.K., and Pecora, P.J., "Outcome Evaluation in Residential Child Care: A Selective North American Review," *Community Care*, in press.

707. Widen, P., "Prospective Payment for Psychiatric Hospitalization: Context and Background," *Hospital and Community Psychiatry* 35(5):447, 1984.

708. Williamson, D.A., Kelley, M.L., Davis, C.J., et al., "Psychopathology of Eating Disorders: A Controlled Comparison of Bulimic, Obese, and Normal Subjects," *Journal of Consulting and Clinical Psychology* 53(2):161, 1985.

709. Wilson, D.R., and Lyman, R.D., "Residential Treatment of Emotionally Disturbed Children," *Handbook of Clinical Child Psychology*, E.C. Walker and M.C. Roberts (eds.) (New York: John Wiley & Sons, 1983).

710. Wiltz, N.A., and Patterson, G.R., "An Evaluation of Parent Training Procedures Designed To Alter Inappropriate Aggressive Behavior of Boys," *Behavior Therapy* 5:215, 1974.

711. Winett, R.A., and Winkler, R.C., "Current Behavior Modification in the Classroom: Be Still, Be Quiet, Be Docile," *Journal of Applied Behavior Analysis* 5:499, 1972.

712. Wing, L., *Early Childhood Autism: Clinical, Educational, and Social Aspects* (Oxford, England: Pergamon Press, 1976).

713. Winokur, G., and Clayton, P., "Family History

Studies: Two Types of Affective Disorders Separated According to Genetic and Clinical Factors," *Recent Advances in Biological Psychiatry*, vol. 9, J. Wortis (ed.) (New York: Plenum Press, 1967).

714. Winsberg, B.G., and Yepes, L.E., "Antipsychotics (Major Tranquilizers, Neuroleptics)," *Pediatric Psychopharmacology: The Use of Behavior Modifying Drugs in Children*, J.S. Werry (ed.) (New York: Brunner/Mazel, 1978).

715. Wolfe, D.A., "Treatment of Abusive Parents: A Reply to the Special Issue," *Journal of Clinical Child Psychiatry* 13(2):192, 1984.

716. Wolpe, J., *Psychotherapy by Reciprocal Inhibition* (Stanford, CA: Stanford University Press, 1958).

717. Worland, J., Edenhart-Pepe, R., Weeks, D.G., et al., "Cognitive Evaluation of Children at Risk: I.Q. Differentiation and Egocentricity," *Children at Risk for Schizophrenia: A Longitudinal Perspective*, N.F. Watt, E.J. Anthony, L.C. Wynne, et al. (eds.) (Cambridge, England: Cambridge University Press, 1984).

718. Worland, J., Jones, C.L., Anthony, E.J., et al., "St. Louis Risk Research Project: Comprehensive Progress Report of Experimental Studies," *Children at Risk for Schizophrenia: A Longitudinal Perspective*, N.F. Watt, E.J. Anthony, L.C. Wynne, et al. (eds.) (Cambridge, England: Cambridge University Press, 1984).

719. Wortman, P., and Saxe, L., "Methods for Evaluating Medical Technology," *Strategies for Medical Assessment*, prepared by the Office of Technology Assessment, U.S. Congress, OTA-H-181 (Washington, DC: U.S. Government Printing Office, September 1982).

720. Wrede, G., Mednick, S.A., Huttunen, M.O., et al., "Pregnancy and Delivery Complications in the Births of an Unselected Series of Finnish Children With Schizophrenic Mothers: II," *Children at Risk for Schizophrenia: A Longitudinal Perspective*, N.F. Watt, E.J. Anthony, L.C. Wynne, et al. (eds.) (Cambridge, England: Cambridge University Press, 1984).

721. Wurtele, S.K., Wilson, D.R., and Prentice-Dunn, S., "Characteristics of Children in Residential Treatment Programs," *Journal of Clinical Child Psychology* 12(2):137, 1983.

722. Yalom, I.D., *The Theory and Practice of Group Psychotherapy* (New York: Basic Books, 1975).

723. Yelton, S., "The Seriously Emotionally Disturbed Juvenile Offender: The Kids Nobody Wants," *Addressing the Mental Health Needs of the Juvenile Justice Population: Policies and Programs*, symposium cosponsored by the National Association of State Mental Health Program Directors and the National Institute of Mental Health, Washington, DC, Feb. 27-28, 1985.

724. Young, T., "Community Mental Health Centers and Their Services for Children and Youth," unpublished paper, University of Chicago School of Social Service Administration, February 1984.

725. Zahn-Waxler, C., McKnew, D.H., Cummings, E.M., et al., "Problem Behaviors and Peer Interactions of Young Children With a Manic-Depressive Parent," *American Journal of Psychiatry* 141(2):236, 1984.

726. Zelnick, M., and Kantner, J.F., "First Pregnancies to Women Aged 15-19: 1976 and 1971," *Family Planning Perspectives* 10:11, 1978.

727. Zigler, E., "Research on Personality Structure of the Retarded," *International Review of Research in Mental Retardation*, N.R. Ellis (ed.) (New York: Academic Press, 1966).

728. Zigler, E., "Assessing Head-Start at 20—and Invited Commentary," *American Journal of Orthopsychiatry* 55(4):603-609, 1985.

729. Zigler, E.F., "Understanding Child Abuse: A Dilemma for Policy Development," *Children, Families, and Government: Perspectives on American Social Policy*, E.F. Zigler, S.L. Kagan, and E. Klugman (eds.) (Cambridge, England: Cambridge University Press, 1983).

730. Zigler, E.F., and Balla, D., "Developmental Course of Responsiveness to Social Reinforcement in Normal Children and Institutionalized Retarded Children," *Developmental Psychology* 6:66, 1972.

731. Zigler, E.F., and Berman, W., "Discerning the Future of Early Childhood Intervention," *American Psychologist* 38:894, 1983.

732. Zigler, E.F., and Child, I.L. (eds.), *Socialization and Personality Development* (Reading, MA: Addison-Wesley, 1973).

733. Zigler, E., and Trickett, P., "I.Q., Social Competence and Evaluation of Early Childhood Intervention Programs," *American Psychologist* 33:789, 1978.

734. Zigler, E.F., and Valentine, J. (eds.), *Project Head Start: A Legacy of the War on Poverty* (New York: Free Press, 1979).

735. Zimet, S.G., and Farley, G.K., "Day Treatment for Children in the United States: An Overview," *Journal of the American Academy of Child Psychiatry*, in press.

736. Zimmerman, J., and Sims, D., "Family Ther-

apy," *Handbook of Clinical Child Psychology*, C.E. Walker and M.C. Roberts (eds.) (New York: John Wiley & Sons, 1983).

737. Zuckerman, K., Ambuel, J., and Bandman, R., "Child Neglect and Abuse: A Study of Cases Evaluated at Columbia Children's Hospital in 1968-1969," *Ohio State Medical Journal* 68:629, 1972.

O